613.90
FOCUS

D1779815

APR '98

613.907 P743f

Poe, Elizabeth Ann.

Focus on sexuality

MAR 3 1 1993		
JUL 0 5 2007		
MAY 2 6 1994		
AUG 9 0 9W		
DEC 1 4 1994		
JAN 2 1 1995		
DEC 04 1995		
JAN 0 2 1996		
MAY 0 3 1996		
AUG 4 2 1999		
DEC 2 7 1999		
FEB 0 1 2001		
JUN 1 9 2001		
JUN 1 2 2001		
	261-2500	Printed in USA

DISCARD

ENTERED DEC 1 5 1992

Focus on
Sexuality

A Reference Handbook

TEENAGE PERSPECTIVES

Focus on Sexuality

A Reference Handbook

Elizabeth Ann Poe
University of Wisconsin–Eau Claire

ABC-CLIO

Santa Barbara, California
Oxford, England

613.907 P743f

Poe, Elizabeth Ann.

Focus on sexuality

© 1990 by ABC-CLIO, Inc.

All rights reserved. No part of this publication may be reproduced, stored in a retrieval system, or transmitted, in any form or by any means, electronic, mechanical, photocopying, recording, or otherwise, except for the inclusion of brief quotations in a review, without prior permission in writing from the publishers.

Library of Congress Cataloging-in-Publication Data
Poe, Elizabeth Ann.
    Focus on sexuality : a reference handbook / Elizabeth Ann Poe.
      p. cm. — (Teenage perspectives)
    Includes bibliographical references and index.
    Summary: Introduces teens to various aspects of sexual development during adolescence, such as physical changes, pregnancy, birth control, and sexually transmitted diseases.
    1. Teenagers—Sexual behavior—Juvenile literature. 2. Sex instruction for teenagers. [1. Sex instruction for youth.]
    I. Title. II. Series.
    HQ27.P64   1990   613.9'07—dc20   90-43661

ISBN 0-87436-116-8 (alk. paper)

97 96 95 94 93 92 91 90   10 9 8 7 6 5 4 3 2 1

ABC-CLIO, Inc.
130 Cremona Drive, P.O. Box 1911
Santa Barbara, California 93116-1911

Clio Press Ltd.
55 St. Thomas' Street
Oxford, OX1 1JG, England

This book is Smyth-sewn and printed on acid-free paper ∞ .
Manufactured in the United States of America

To Ruth

Contents

Foreword, xi

Preface, xiii

Acknowledgments, xv

Chapter 1: Sexuality, 1

What Is Sexuality?, 2
How Is Sexuality Shaped?, 2
Expressions of Sexuality, 3
Sexual Activities, 4
Sexual Orientation, 6
Values and Choices, 8

Resources for Finding Out about Sexuality, 12
Sexuality in Fiction, 12
Nonfiction Materials on Sexuality, 20
Nonprint Materials on Sexuality, 23
Organizations Concerned with Teen Sexuality, 33
Hotline, 35

Chapter 2: Physical Development, 37

Male and Female Reproductive Systems, 38
Sexual Intercourse for Reproduction, 41
Sexual Development, 42
Emotions Accompanying Sexual Development, 46

Resources for Finding Out about Physical Development, 49
Physical Development in Fiction, 49

Nonfiction Materials on Physical Development, 50
Nonprint Materials on Physical Development, 52
Organizations Concerned with Physical Development and
    Related Issues, 54

Chapter 3: Contraception, 57

Contraceptives: To Use or Not To Use, 58
Birth-Control Methods, 61
Fallacies about Birth Control, 77
Conclusion, 77

Resources for Finding Out about Contraception, 79
Contraception in Fiction, 79
Nonfiction Materials on Contraception, 81
Nonprint Materials on Contraception, 84
Organizations Concerned with Contraception, 88

Chapter 4: Teenage Pregnancy, 91

Recognizing Pregnancy, 92
Emotional Responses to Pregnancy, 94
Choices, 95
Other Concerns, 106
Conclusion, 108

Resources for Finding Out about Teenage Pregnancy, 110
Teenage Pregnancy in Fiction, 110
Nonfiction Materials on Teenage Pregnancy, 117
Nonprint Materials on Teenage Pregnancy, 123
Organizations Concerned with Teenage Pregnancy, 132
Hotline, 134

Chapter 5: Sexually Transmitted Diseases, 135

What Is an STD?, 138
Signs of STDs, 138
When an STD Is Suspected, 139
Tests When No Symptoms Are Present, 140
Responsibilities, 140
Types of STDs, 142
Conclusion, 156

Resources for Finding Out about Sexually Transmitted Diseases, 158
Sexually Transmitted Diseases in Fiction, 158
Nonfiction Materials on Sexually Transmitted Diseases, 160
Nonprint Materials on Sexually Transmitted Diseases, 167
Organizations Concerned with Sexually Transmitted Diseases, 177
Hotlines, 178

Chapter 6: Unwanted Sexual Contact, 183

Sexual Assault, 185
Sexual Abuse, 192
Help for Victims of Unwanted Sexual Contact, 195

Resources for Finding Out about Unwanted Sexual Contact, 197
Unwanted Sexual Contact in Fiction, 197
Nonfiction Materials on Unwanted Sexual Contact, 201
Nonprint Materials on Unwanted Sexual Contact, 206
Organizations Concerned with Unwanted Sexual Contact, 210
Hotline, 211

Index, 213

Foreword

An old Chinese curse goes, "May you live in exciting times." Today's young people have grown up under such a curse—or blessing. They live in a world that is undergoing dramatic changes on every level—social, political, scientific, environmental, technological. At the same time, while still in school, they are dealing with serious issues, making choices and confronting dilemmas that previous generations never dreamed of.

Technology, especially telecommunications and computers, has made it possible for young people to know a great deal about their world and what goes on in it, at least on a surface level. They have access to incredible amounts of information, yet much of that information seems irrelevant to their daily lives. When it comes to grappling with the issues that actually touch them, they may have a tough time finding out what they need to know.

The Teenage Perspectives series is designed to give young people access to information on the topics that are closest to their lives or that deeply concern them—topics like families, school, health, sexuality, and drug abuse. Having knowledge about these issues can make it easier to understand and cope with them, and to make appropriate and beneficial choices. The books can be used as tools for researching school assignments, or for finding out about topics of personal concern. Adults who are working with young people, such as teachers, counselors, librarians, and parents, will also find these books useful. Many of the references cited can be used for planning information or discussion sessions with adults as well as young people.

Ruth K. J. Cline
Series Editor

Preface

Adolescence is a time of discovering and defining one's identity, and sexuality plays an important role in this process. Teenagers are naturally curious as they observe their bodies developing and their feelings changing. They have many questions about their own sexual development and how sexuality is expressed. They may have friends they wish to help or better understand. They also want to know how to protect themselves in a time when sexual contact can cause problems.

Focus on Sexuality: A Reference Handbook is designed to help answer teens' questions about sexuality. Each chapter provides basic information on an aspect of sexuality of particular interest to teens. Although sexuality is not a topic of interest only to teenagers, the information provided here is tailored to adolescents.

Chapter 1 examines what is meant by sexuality, focusing on how it is shaped and expressed. Chapter 2 describes the physical developments taking place during adolescence. Chapter 3 explains the various forms of contraception and the facts to consider when deciding on contraceptive use. Chapter 4 looks at teen pregnancy and the options involved. Chapter 5 describes different types of sexually transmitted diseases and ways to prevent their spread. Chapter 6 discusses various types of unwanted sexual contact and how to handle these situations.

The Resources section included in each chapter contains annotated lists of fiction, nonfiction, and nonprint materials, as well as hotlines and organizations related to the chapter topic. In the listings of books, paperback publishers are indicated in parentheses.

The selection criteria for these sources included accuracy, readability, accessibility, and timeliness. Fiction books listed are young-adult novels, written for junior and senior high school students. Most of these novels have recent copyright dates, but some older books are included either to provide perspective and background on the topic or because they have become standard fare for these topics. A number of these books address topics from one or more chapters. Except in the case of teenage pregnancy books, books are listed in each chapter to which they apply with the relevant aspects spotlighted in the annotation.

Nonfiction entries are primarily books, but some journals and pamphlets are included. For the most part, nonfiction materials were written for or are appropriate reading for junior and senior high students. Notes are made in the annotations to signal difficult reading or information levels.

Highly technical sources, like government documents, may be used in the chapter and listed as references, but are not necessarily annotated in the Resources sections. Materials were selected to present a balanced view of the topic. As in the case of fiction books, nonfiction materials are cross-referenced in the various chapters with relevant aspects highlighted in the annotations.

Nonprint materials, primarily films and videocassettes, were selected from a wealth of possibilities. Selection criteria focused on applicability to a teenage audience.

Sources of help from organizations are included at the end of each chapter. Information about national organizations is provided, and, in the case of sexually transmitted diseases, state hotlines are also listed. Some organizations offer personal help and others give general information or serve as referral agencies.

Acknowledgments

I would like to thank Judith Volc, Tracy Wahl, Larry Hale, and Lynette Perrault for their assistance in the research aspects of this manuscript, and my husband, Larry Oakes (a nice guy!), for his technical assistance. I would also like to pay tribute to my former students at the Jefferson County (Colorado) Teen Mother Program and thank them for providing me, as an adult, with a window into teenage sexuality.

CHAPTER 1

Sexuality

"Yes," Mrs. Fulton agreed. "Our sexual feelings and our sexual behavior are very private parts of who we are." She agreed, but it didn't stop her from talking about it.
>Jenny Davis, *Sex Education* (New York: Orchard Books, 1988), 10.

"I was wondering about gay people," I said quickly. "Actually, I was wondering about regular—I mean heterosexual people who think about things gay people do. Like a heterosexual guy thinking about another guy that way," I said. What a muddle.

"Oh, you mean heterosexuals who have homosexual fantasies?"

That was easy enough, I thought, a little relieved. Does she know why I'm asking? She must.

"Yeah," I continued. "I mean—is it sick?"

"Not at all. It's normal, as a matter of fact."

"It is?"

"Sure. A lot of people probably do become sexually attracted to someone of their own sex at one time or another."

Sexually *attracted*—so that's what my daydreams mean, I thought.
>Deborah Hautzig, *Hey, Dollface* (New York: Greenwillow Books, 1978), 111–112.

In these passages, taken from novels written for young adults, teenagers are discussing sexuality with high school teachers. In the first novel, *Sex Education*, 14-year-old Olivia Sinclair is studying sex education in Mrs. Fulton's biology class. Mrs. Fulton is just starting to discuss why some people are shy or embarrassed when talking about sexuality. In the second novel, *Hey, Dollface*, 16-year-old Valerie Hoffman is indirectly asking Miss Udry whether she is a lesbian because she has sexual fantasies about her best friend, Chleo. Both these teens show normal curiosity about the general nature of sexuality and their own developing sexual awareness.

What Is Sexuality?

Sexuality involves so many aspects it is difficult to define, but since it is such an important part of being human, it deserves serious consideration. A person's sexuality is based on his or her feelings about being a male or a female (either individually or as a member of a group), his or her feelings about the opposite sex, and his or her feelings about engaging in activities that express how it feels to be a male or a female. The physical differences between the bodies of males and females are part of our sexuality, but so is the socialization each of us receives based on these differences and on perceived sex role expectations. Some aspects of sexuality, therefore, are innate, or inborn, while other aspects are determined by the environment into which we are born.

How Is Sexuality Shaped?

From the time we are born, we start to develop and express our sexuality. Babies seem to experience sexual sensations as they respond pleasurably when they discover and fondle their own genitals or cuddle up to a mother's breast. Children thrive as parents express their love for them with hugs and kisses. Adolescents experience hormonal and physical changes that often intensify those feelings that are in any way associated with the fact that they are male or female. These sexual sensations are part of our sexuality and underlie our general functioning as sexual beings.

But sexuality is not only physical. Sexuality also includes what we think and how we behave. Sexuality involves how a teenage girl believes she should act because she is a female. Much of her sexuality will be a response to how her mother behaves, or how her father treats her, or what her brothers say about her. The same is true for adolescent boys.

Society also influences our sexuality, by indicating that boys and girls should behave in particular ways. The mass-communications media project certain images of sexuality that many people try to adopt. For example, men are frequently portrayed as muscular, athletic, aggressive, and competitive; women are slim, beautiful, passive, and nurturing. Some people accept these stereotypes without thinking about them; other people think about them and decide what parts of these images to accept and what to reject. In this way they are shaping their own sexuality.

Expressions of Sexuality

People express their sexuality through talking, laughing, kissing, touching, dancing, painting, writing, sculpting, or any of the other ways individuals communicate what they are feeling as male and female human beings. Sexuality can involve touching without implying sexual desire. For example, people often put an arm around someone who is suffering. This is a show of concern, not a sexual come-on.

Of course, sexuality is often related to the type of touching connected with sexual stimulation and arousal. This type of sexual contact elicits certain physical responses.

When a boy is sexually aroused, his penis may harden into an erection. Girls may secrete extra fluid in the vaginal area when they are sexually aroused. These normal responses to sexual stimulation may go away, or they may continue to build to a climax during which the excitement becomes intensely pleasurable and the built-up sexual tension is released through orgasm. At the time of orgasm, the boy ejaculates.

Following orgasm, the boy's or girl's body then returns to a relaxed, unstimulated state in which the penis becomes soft, or flaccid, and the girl's vagina stops secreting lubricating fluid.

Sexual arousal does not have to climax in orgasm, however. If the stimulation stops, the sexually aroused person gradually relaxes, and his or her body returns to an unaroused state.

Sexual Activities

People can be sexually aroused by many types of activities and situations. They can be sexually aroused by an idea or a fantasy, the proximity of a sexually attractive person, or a number of other occurrences. They can be aroused when they are alone or with another. Some of the sexual activities in which humans engage include masturbation, kissing, making out, petting, and sexual intercourse.

MASTURBATION

Masturbation means stimulating one's own or another's genitals for the purpose of achieving orgasm without involving sexual intercourse. Most medical professionals consider masturbation to be a normal, natural, and healthy activity in which people engage throughout their lifetimes.

- "The vast majority of Americans of both sexes and all ages masturbate, giving themselves pleasure and releasing sexual tensions" (Hein, 243).

Besides giving pleasure and releasing tensions, masturbating enables people to explore various aspects of their sexuality without risking pregnancy or sexually transmitted diseases.

The numerous myths about the consequences of masturbating are not true. Masturbation does not cause blindness, baldness, acne, madness, or any of the other ill effects attributed to it. Some religious groups oppose masturbation because it is a sexual activity that does not create children. Some adults teach children it is wrong to touch their genitals. Teens with these kinds of upbringing may feel uncomfortable or guilty when they masturbate. While masturbating is considered by many people to be a normal activity, it is certainly not abnormal if one chooses not to masturbate.

KISSING

Some people may feel discomfort about masturbation, but kissing a sexually attractive person is generally considered a pleasurable experience. To many people, kissing is a first and important step in a sexual encounter. When people French-kiss, they open their mouths so their tongues can touch and/or enter the other person's mouth. This is sometimes called open-mouth or deep kissing.

MAKING OUT

Making out is a sexual activity involving intense kissing, hugging, and rubbing of the back. These activities can continue for long periods of time, during which couples become very excited and stimulated.

PETTING

When sexual activities move from kissing and making out to include the boy feeling the girl's breasts, either through her bra or under it, the couple is now involved in petting. Sometimes this intense contact includes touching or rubbing against each other's genitals. Sometimes couples choose to mutually masturbate and give each other an orgasm. Couples can reach orgasms through manual masturbation or by rubbing against each other's genitals, with or without their clothes on. Many couples find petting to be a very satisfying sexual experience.

SEXUAL INTERCOURSE

Kissing, making out, petting—these are all sexual activities that vary in their intensity and that may or may not lead to sexual intercourse, or going all the way, as it is often called. When they do lead to intercourse, they are referred to as foreplay.

Sexual intercourse, also just called sex, is defined as an intimate physical relationship involving use of the sex organs, which are the penis and the vagina (see Chapter 2). When the penis is inserted into the vagina, the activity is called vaginal intercourse. Inserting the penis into the mouth or stimulating the vagina with the mouth is called oral sex. Inserting the penis into the anus is called anal sex. Each of these types of sex involves the same pattern of sexual response described earlier.

Sexual intercourse is only one type of sexual activity. Many teens do not feel they are ready for or want to engage in sexual intercourse, but this does not mean they cannot engage in other sexual activities. People enjoy different types of sexual activities during different times in their lives and at different points in their relationships with other people. A person's age or sexual orientation can have a great deal to do with the type of sexual activities he or she likes or chooses.

Sexual Orientation

Part of sexuality involves being attracted to other people. Attractions may be emotional, intellectual, spiritual, sexual, or a combination of these.

Adolescents often admire an older person of the same sex, and may feel strongly attracted to him or her for some special reason. For example, a teenage girl may admire a female teacher (or doctor or architect or artist) because she is intellectually stimulating as well as a successful wife and mother. The girl may feel a special attraction to this woman because she is leading the type of full life the girl herself hopes to lead one day. In this situation, the teacher's gender is important because she is a sex role model for the student. Sexuality is involved, even though the attraction is not sexual.

Of course, the primary focus of some relationships is sexual attraction, and these can have several different orientations.

HETEROSEXUALITY

Heterosexual comes from Greek word parts that mean having to do with the opposite sex. People who are heterosexually oriented are generally sexually attracted to the opposite sex. Most of American society is geared toward this heterosexual, or straight, orientation, and other approaches to sexuality are commonly misunderstood. Heterosexual activities include all those described earlier.

HOMOSEXUALITY

Homosexuality, from the Greek words that mean having to do with the same sex, is a sexual orientation that some adolescents embrace temporarily, while for others it is a lifelong preference.

- Seventeen percent of American males aged 16 to 19 have had one or more homosexual experiences (Hein, 242).
- Six percent of American females aged 16 to 19 have had homosexual experiences (ibid.).
- Ten percent of the adult population is made up of homosexuals (Heron, 7).

The term gay refers to all homosexuals. Female homosexuals are also called lesbians.

Many adult homosexuals say they knew at a young age that they were attracted to people of their same sex. However, because of misunderstandings about and prejudices toward homosexuals, they had to mask their sexuality and pretend to be heterosexual.

When gay people tell their friends or society in general that they are homosexual, it is called coming out, referring to the action as "coming out of the closet" and expressing their sexuality openly. It is important to note that "homosexuality is natural and normal for a minority of the population of any country, and has been since earliest recorded history" (Hein, 242). Homosexual activities include all those described earlier with the exception of vaginal intercourse.

BISEXUALITY

Some people are not completely homosexual or heterosexual and are sexually attracted to both the same and the opposite sex. They are called bisexuals because *bi* is the Greek word part meaning two. These are usually not people who may have had a few homosexual experiences in their early years, but rather those who have no preference for one sex over the other. Bisexual activities include all the sexual activities described earlier.

TRANSSEXUALS

While heterosexuals, homosexuals, and bisexuals see and identify themselves as male or female according to their anatomies, transsexuals see themselves as the opposite sex. Male transsexuals, for example, psychologically identify with females, and see themselves as women, not men. Transsexuals sometimes undergo surgery to change their sex. If a sex change occurs, they would be able to engage in vaginal sex.

TRANSVESTITES

Transvestites are homosexual or heterosexual people who enjoy behaving as and dressing in the clothing of the opposite sex.

Values and Choices

So far, much of this chapter has described the physical side of sexuality. But, as was mentioned earlier, sexuality also involves feelings and thoughts. Sexuality involves making choices, and choices involve values. Values help people determine what is acceptable or unacceptable behavior, or what they should and should not do.

Adolescence is a time when many people develop their personal value systems. Personal values usually do not exist in isolation; they are shaped by families, friends, churches, schools, communities, and society. From birth, teenagers watch what others do and hear what others advise; these observations influence the values they develop for themselves.

When developing their sexual values, some teens completely accept the guidance of their parents or religious community, embracing those teachings as their own. Other teens rebel, rejecting whatever their parents, school personnel, and/or religious leaders say. Some teens accept the values of their peer group without much question. Others choose to consider various perspectives as they develop their own sexual values.

In any case, everyone has behaviors he or she feels are important and desirable. When people say a teenager has no values, what they are really saying is that the teen's values differ from their own values. Generally speaking, if a person's values do not hurt that person, other people, or society at large, most people will respect an individual's right to uphold his or her own values. When it comes to sexual matters, it is often difficult to make decisions that do not hurt anyone. That's why sexual choices must be carefully considered. Some questions to think about might include:

> How do I want to express my sexuality?
>
> What does sex mean to me?
>
> What does sex mean to my partner (or date, or boyfriend, or girlfriend)?
>
> Should sex involve love?
>
> Do I want to become sexually active while I am a teenager?
>
> What would I like my first sexual experience to be like?
>
> If I have sex once, can I ever say no again?
>
> How do I want my sexual partner to treat me?
>
> How do I want to treat my sexual partner?

Do I want to wait until I am married to have sex?
Will I use a method of birth control?
How will I protect against sexually transmitted diseases?
Is it important to talk about sex with my sexual partner?
What does my religious upbringing say about sex and sexuality?
What would I do if I became pregnant?
What would I do if my girlfriend became pregnant?
What are my family's views about sex?
Do I want to have many sexual partners in my lifetime, or few, or only one?
Is it okay for boys to have lots of sexual experiences but not okay for girls?
What will I do if others try to pressure me to do something I don't want to?
Which of my friends have values I agree with?
What types of sexual activities do I feel comfortable with?

These questions have to do with sexual values and choices. Most of them are not easy to answer. And there are, of course, many more. The text in this book is written to provide some general information that may be useful when a teenager is thinking about questions like these. The resources listed at the end of each chapter provide more detailed information, opinions, and, in some cases, advice about sexuality.

Sexuality is a complex phenomenon. Most people are naturally curious about this fascinating, complex, and important part of human behavior.

REFERENCES

Bell, Ruth, et al. *Changing Bodies, Changing Lives: A Book for Teens on Sex and Relationships.* New York: Random House, 1987.

Davis, Jenny. *Sex Education.* New York: Orchard Books, 1988.

Eagan, Andrea Boroff. *Why Am I So Miserable If These Are the Best Years of My Life?* New York: Avon, 1988.

Hautzig, Deborah. *Hey, Dollface*. New York: Greenwillow Books, 1978.

Hein, Karen. "Adolescence and Sexual Maturity." In *The Columbia University College of Physicians and Surgeons Complete Home Medical Guide*, ed. Donald F. Tapley, et al., 231–256. Mt. Vernon, NY: Consumers Union, 1985.

Heron, Ann, ed. *One Teenager in Ten: Writings by Gay and Lesbian Youth*. Boston: Alyson Publications, 1983.

Johnson, Eric W. *Love & Sex in Plain Language*. New York: Bantam, 1988.

Madaras, Lynda, with Area Madaras. *The What's Happening to My Body? Book for Girls: A Growing Up Guide for Parents and Daughters*. New York: Newmarket Press, 1988.

Madaras, Lynda, with Dane Saavedra. *The What's Happening to My Body? Book for Boys: A Growing Up Guide for Parents and Sons*. New York: Newmarket Press, 1987.

McCoy, Kathy, and Charles Wibbelsman. *The New Teenage Body Book*. Los Angeles: Body Press, 1984.

Resources
for Finding Out about Sexuality

Sexuality in Fiction

This section contains a list of novels written specifically for young adults about subjects involving sexuality. Although books on dating and romance also involve sexuality, they are not included here. In addition, books primarily about teenage pregnancy, although they also involve teen sexuality, are not included here. They can be found in the resources section in Chapter 4.

The titles listed here address or mention topics such as sexual decision making, premarital sex, masturbation, and homosexuality. They include earlier as well as recent books dealing with these topics.

Adler, C. S. **Binding Ties.** New York: Delacorte (Dell), 1985. 183p.

Sixteen-year-old Anne is having a passionate love affair with Kyle, but her family, consisting of her mother, grandmother, and aunt, thinks Kyle is too wild for a nice, sensible girl like Anne. Anne feels suffocated by her family's love and exhilarated by Kyle's. When Anne agrees to run away to Arizona with Kyle, her stepsister tells Anne's family, and they try to talk her out of it. When Anne's grandmother breaks her leg, Anne stays to help her while Kyle goes to Arizona by himself. Three weeks later as planned, Anne flies to Arizona, only to find Kyle is living with an older woman, his boss at the gas station. She returns home to the love of her family.

Betancourt, Jeanne. **Sweet Sixteen and Never** ... New York: Bantam, 1987. 136p.

Julie has just turned 16 when she starts dating Sam Stewart. Sam is much more sexually experienced than Julie, who is a virgin, but he takes it very slowly with her. Sam and Julie finally discuss sex and Julie discovers Sam had another experience where the sexual part of the relationship went too fast. Everyone found out and the relationship didn't work. Furthermore, he developed a reputation for helping girls lose their virginity, so girls started to use him.

Sam does not want his relationship with Julie to be this way, so he does not pressure her and wants to wait until they are both ready to have sex. The story ends with this understanding between them.

Blume, Judy. **Forever.** Scarsdale, NY: Bradbury (Pocket Books), 1975. 220p.

This is a classic book about teenage sexuality. Katherine and Michael start going together in the second half of their senior year. Michael is more sexually experienced than Katherine— he has had intercourse twice with a casual acquaintance. He and Katherine decide they would like to have sex, but they take it slowly. Michael assures Katherine that there are no rights and wrongs when it comes to making love. Together, they discover the pleasures of love and sex as they explore their own sexuality. Michael and Katherine vow to love each other forever.

Katherine's parents are concerned about the intensity of her relationship with Michael, and arrange for her to teach tennis lessons at a summer camp. There Katherine meets Theo, whom she finds attractive. Confused by her feelings, Katherine tries to discuss the subject with Michael, but he feels betrayed and breaks up with her.

In a subplot, Katherine's friend Erica becomes interested in Michael's friend Artie. Artie thinks he may be gay and Erica tries to help him discover he is not, but her efforts fail. When Artie's parents forbid him to go to acting school, he attempts suicide and is institutionalized. Erica decides she should not be in such a rush to lose her virginity and sees the value of waiting for love before she experiences sex.

Bograd, Larry. **Travelers.** New York: Lippincott, 1986. 184p.

Jack Karlstad accepts an invitation from his wealthy friend Wendell to drive with him on a long weekend from Colorado to California. Wendell's main objective is to have a good time and lose his virginity, but Jack takes the opportunity to seek out men who knew his father in Vietnam. Jack and Wendell are unsuccessful in their attempt to patronize a brothel, and their dates with two California "valley girls" are equally disappointing. Upon his return home, Jack decides to use the money set aside for his college education to help his grandfather save their family farm. Jack's girlfriend, Brenda, forgives him for his inconsiderateness and volunteers to help him with the farm.

Bridgers, Sue Ellen. **Permanent Connections.** New York: Harper & Row (Harper Keypoint), 1987. 264p.

Rob is forced to leave his plush city life and care for his uncle in a small mountain village in North Carolina. There he meets Ellery, another outsider forced away from the city life. They make love spontaneously one afternoon, but argue afterward when Rob wants to do it again. Rob thinks protection from disease is all they need to worry about, but Ellery wants to talk about their feelings. Rob deals with his frustration by getting drunk.

   Ellery discovers that her cousin, Leanna, and her boyfriend, Travis, are sexually active. Rob gets in trouble with drugs; his grandfather is seriously injured; and Rob begins to understand the meaning of family love and support.

Davis, Jenny. **Sex Education.** New York: Orchard Books, 1988. 150p.

Olivia (Livvie) Sinclair and David Kindler are ninth-grade students taking Biology 200 from Mrs. Fulton. The first semester of the course is sex education, but not by the book. Mrs. Fulton is trying to teach about the physiology of sex and the emotional aspects of sexuality. The students are assigned to think about sex, to look at their own bodies, and to care about someone. Livvie and David do all their assignments successfully, and the one about caring changes them forever.

Garden, Nancy. **Annie on My Mind.** New York: Farrar, Straus & Giroux, 1982. 234p.

Liza, a senior at a coed private school, develops a close friendship with Annie, a junior at the public high school. When their relationship becomes physical, they realize they are gay. They want a place where they can be alone to express the physical part of their love. When Liza volunteers to feed the cats of two teachers who share an apartment, Annie and Liza find out these teachers are lesbians.

The girls' homosexual relationship is discovered by school officials, and in the course of the proceedings, the homosexual teachers are fired. Liza, afraid of hurting her supportive mother, lies and says she and Annie never did more than hug and kiss. The following year Liza, now a college student, calls Annie and tells her she loves her.

Guy, Rosa. **Ruby.** New York: Viking (Bantam), 1976. 217p.

This is the story of a love affair between Ruby and Daphne. Ruby, 18, has recently immigrated from the West Indies to Harlem. Her mother has recently died, her father is overbearing, and her sister has withdrawn into the world of books. Ruby is desperately lonely and finds solace in the friendship of the cool, beautiful, intelligent Daphne. Their friendship grows into a full-fledged love affair that ends sadly when Daphne decides Ruby is not right for her.

Hall, Lynn. **Sticks and Stones.** New York: Follett (Dell), 1972. 197p.

Tom, a brilliant pianist, is told he cannot attend the state music competition because the townspeople believe he is a homosexual. Although the accusation is false, and based on a rumor started by two insecure schoolmates, Tom starts to doubt his masculinity. Tom's friend Ward finally tells him the rumor started because Ward was discharged from the service for having a homosexual encounter.

Although Tom initially cuts himself off from Ward, he later realizes he has become self-destructive. Tom learns to ignore the whispers and not allow other people to tell him who he is. Although this book involves the issue of homosexuality and provides some useful information about the topic, it is really about gossip, small-mindedness, revenge, and belief in oneself.

Hautzig, Deborah. **Hey, Dollface.** New York: Greenwillow Books (Bantam), 1978. 151p.

Valerie Hoffman and Chleo Fox are the best of friends. They enjoy talking, painting, and skipping school together; they would rather be together than with anyone else. Val has sexual fantasies about Chleo and realizes she is sexually attracted to Chleo. Val feels guilty and confused. She talks to her mother and a teacher about general sexual concerns, but is not able to discuss her feelings with Chleo. One night they have a mild homosexual experience. Several weeks later, they talk about their feelings. Both girls acknowledge their love for each other as well as their ability to be attracted to the opposite sex. They appreciate the wonderful complexity of their relationship.

Holland, Isabelle. **The Man without a Face.** Philadelphia: Lippincott (Bantam), 1972. 151p.

Fourteen-year-old Chuck Norstadt needs a tutor to help him pass the entrance exams for boarding school. Justin McLeod, a recluse with a severely scarred face, reluctantly agrees to tutor Chuck and proves to be a demanding teacher. Chuck and Justin are attracted to one another and have a brief homosexual encounter. Chuck is initially angry and upset, but later comes to understand the meaning of love, friendship, and compassion.

Kerr, M. E. **Night Kites.** New York: Harper & Row (Harper Keypoint), 1986. 216p.

High school senior Erick Rudd can't believe how lucky he is to be having a passionate love affair with the exotic Nicki. Not only is Nicki helping him explore his sexuality, she is also helping take his mind off his home situation.

Klein, Norma. **Angel Face.** New York: Fawcett Juniper, 1984. 245p.

Angel Face is the story of a boy, Jason, 16. At the same time that his parents are getting a divorce, Jason is starting his first "real" relationship with a girl, Vicki. As Vicki and Jason explore their sexuality, each shows great respect for the other. Jason does not push Vicki to greater limits, although he would like to. Vicki understands Jason's anxiety after his mother dies, and she does not push him. It is a story about showing respect for the feelings of others.

Jason's older brother, Tyler, is his role model. After watching the relationship between Ty and Juliet develop and then fall apart, Jason sees exactly what not to do. This book realistically explores the feelings of two teenagers who are experiencing their first love and how they grow to understand each other, themselves, and their feelings about sexuality.

Koertge, Ron. **The Arizona Kid.** Boston: Little, Brown, 1988. 228p.

Billy leaves his family and friends in Bradyville, Missouri, and spends the summer in Arizona, living with his gay uncle and working at a racetrack. Billy is delighted to be a cowboy, complete with hat and boots, but he learns about much more than horses. He gains insight into the gay lifestyle of his uncle. He also falls in love with Cara Mae, and they share their first sexual experience and explore their sexuality together. This book is not only insightful and informative, but is also very funny and delightful to read.

Koertge, Ron. **Where the Kissing Never Stops.** Boston: Little, Brown (Dell), 1986. 224p.

This story of first love, told by 17-year-old Walker, gives a male perspective on teenage romance. The bad news is that Walker's father has recently died, and his mother has taken a job as a stripper. The good news is that Walker and Rachel really like each other and share their first sexual experiences together. In an open, honest relationship, they discuss their feelings about their own bodies. Walker's wonderful sense of humor runs throughout the book as he describes his cravings for junk food, his erections, his masturbating, and his loss of innocence. But he has a genuine reverence for the mysteriousness of sex and his feelings about Rachel.

Mazer, Harry. **The Girl of His Dreams.** New York: Crowell (Avon), 1987. 214p.

Eighteen-year-old Willis Pierce dreams of the perfect girl. Straight from the farm, 22-year-old Sophie is definitely not his dream girl, but she turns out be just what he needs. They talk about their feelings and hopes; they laugh and argue; and eventually they become lovers. Willis learns the importance of considering Sophie's feelings because he now has someone to love.

Mazer, Harry. **I Love You, Stupid.** New York: Crowell (Flare), 1981. 185p.

Lusty sexual fantasies abound for high school senior Marcus Rosenbloom, but he cannot manage to climb the wall that separates the sexually experienced from the inexperienced. Then his childhood friend Wendy Barrett moves back into town. Marcus and Wendy develop a friendship that includes a lot of joking, arguing, hanging out, and talking about the perplexities and frustrations of sex and male-female relationships. As friends, they decide to help each other into the world of the sexually experienced. There they discover more than just sex and friendship—they find love. Mazer portrays the male point of view perceptively (including masturbation) while maintaining a humorous tone.

Mazer, Norma Fox. **Up in Seth's Room.** New York: Delacorte (Dell), 1979. 199p.

Finn is madly in love with Seth, but her parents forbid her to see him. Not only is Seth the brother of the man their other daughter is living with against their will, but he is also 19 and Finn is 15. Finn knows her own mind about sex. She feels she is too young and it's too important, but she finds Seth terribly exciting. She sees him first against her parents' wishes and then openly, although they still do not approve.

Seth does not believe Finn when she says she does not want to have sex, and he tries to pressure her into it. She refuses and they fight. Later they talk it over, and he realizes they can love each other without having sex. Finn learns to reach orgasm without having intercourse. She and Seth part when he goes to work on a farm in Vermont, but their experience has made them both grow and understand the power of love and sexual expression.

Scoppettone, Sandra. **Happy Endings Are All Alike.** New York: Harper & Row (Dell), 1978. 202p.
Jaret and Peggy, recent high school graduates, have been lovers for several months. Although they are not ashamed of their relationship, few people know they are lesbians. Peggy is not as sure of her homosexuality as is Jaret, and after Jaret is raped, Peggy asks her not to press charges and expose their relationship to the whole town. Jaret does anyway and after a month's separation and sessions with a psychiatrist, Peggy learns about herself and realizes she loves Jaret. The two reunite, knowing there are no certainties for the future, only happy moments. This book provides insight into many facets of a relationship between young lesbians.

Strasser, Todd. **A Very Touchy Subject.** New York: Delacorte (Dell), 1985. 181p.
Seventeen-year-old Scott Tauscher figures he spends 47 percent of each day, on the average, thinking about sex. However, Alix Shuman, his girlfriend of two years, refuses even to discuss the subject, and they break up. His next-door neighbor, 15-year-old Paula Finkel, on the other hand, has a boyfriend who sneaks out of her window every morning. Scott learns that Paula's mother is an alcoholic who abuses Paula. Paula lets her boyfriend have sex, even though she knows he's using her, because she needs to feel close to someone.

Scott drives Paula to her father in North Carolina. They have car trouble and are forced to spend the night in his van. Paula offers herself to Scott, but he says no because he knows Paula wants to change her ways and his taking advantage would not help her. Scott forgoes his golden opportunity to lose his virginity, but he knows he's done the right thing.

Williams, Grace. **The Very Last Virgin at Hobeck High.** New York: Signet, 1986. 157p.

Everyone in Annie's high school seems to be pressuring her into sex. She is known to all as The Virgin. She hears girls talking about her in the locker room, and a boy offers to take care of her little problem if she will switch his picture in the yearbook. She really wants to lose this title, but she wants it to be with the right person. When she finds the right boy, she discovers he is also a virgin. They decide together that they are not ready for sex just yet. Annie, therefore, decides to withstand the pressure her schoolmates are putting upon her.

Zindel, Bonnie. **Hollywood Dream Machine.** New York: Viking (Bantam), 1984. 179p.

Gabrielle Fuller, 17, spends the summer with her best friend, Buffy, whose family has moved from New York to California. Caught up in the fast-paced California lifestyle, Gabrielle instantly falls in love with Bradley Randolph (Bear), who is handsome and wealthy—her perfect prince. Bear's invitation to spend the night with him in a hotel forces Gabrielle to grapple with her emotions and values. She decides she is not yet ready for sex. Angry at first, Bear tells her their relationship is over, but he later apologizes. He learns that he admires her convictions, and they decide to work on developing their relationship. Gabrielle learns that, to be truly free, she must think for herself, even if it means risking losing the one she loves.

Nonfiction Materials on Sexuality

The following books contain information about teenage sexuality. Some of them are about a specific topic pertaining to sexuality, but most of them are comprehensive resources that contain information about many aspects of sexuality. The aspects relevant to this chapter are highlighted in these annotations.

Bell, Ruth, et al. **Changing Bodies, Changing Lives: A Book for Teens on Sex and Relationships.** New York: Random House, 1987. 254p.

This comprehensive book includes information on all aspects of teen sexuality and general health. It was written specifically for teenagers. Teens from across the country were consulted about its contents, and they share their views on their own sexuality and sexual experiences. The authors write in a straightforward manner and provide a range of perspectives on each topic. This is one of the best resources available for teens.

Eagan, Andrea Boroff. **Why Am I So Miserable If These Are the Best Years of My Life?: Everything Your Mother Never Told You about Becoming a Woman.** New York: Avon, 1988. 211p.

Eagan stresses being yourself and making your own decisions. She discusses many topics including sexual stereotypes and changing sex roles; pressures from friends, society, and the commercial world; and sex. Her style is straightforward and her information is factual. She adds her own opinions at times. Her background in the women's liberation and women's health movements is evident in this frank, honest, readable guide for young women.

Heron, Ann, ed. **One Teenager in Ten: Writings by Gay and Lesbian Youth.** Boston: Alyson, 1983. 115p.

In this book 26 homosexuals, ranging from age 15 to 24, from all parts of the United States and two from Canada, write about their coming-out experiences. Their stories portray the joy, sadness, fear, anger, confusion, acceptance, and pride they feel, and provide the reader with some sense of what it is like to be young and gay today. Some of the authors address their remarks to teens who have not fully accepted their homosexuality. Others give names of books and/or organizations that helped them accept their gayness.

Johnson, Eric W. **Love & Sex in Plain Language.** Philadelphia: Lippincott (Bantam), 1985. 207p.

Originally written in 1968, this is the fourth revision of this comprehensive but concise book. In addition to other topics, the author discusses homosexuality, ways that sex can be a problem, and sexual decision making. Along with factual information, Johnson offers a framework of values to guide people in making decisions involving sex and love. This book is not difficult to read. Illustrations, a glossary, and an index make the information readily accessible.

Madaras, Lynda, with Area Madaras. **The What's Happening to My Body? Book for Girls: A Growing Up Guide for Parents and Daughters.** New York: Newmarket, 1988. 269p.

This book was written especially for younger adolescents and their parents by a leading sex educator and her teenage daughter. Although the primary focus is female puberty, the topics of sexual feelings and sexual intercourse are also discussed, but not in as much detail. The frank, clear explanations and conversational writing style make the information accessible to the intended audience. Illustrations enhance the text, and an index is included.

Madaras, Lynda, with Dane Saavedra. **The What's Happening to My Body? Book for Boys: A Growing Up Guide for Parents and Sons.** New York: Newmarket, 1987. 251p.

Written by a leading sex educator with the assistance of a teenage boy, this book deals primarily with male puberty. Brief information about sexual feelings and sexual intercourse is included. The tone is honest and conversational. The intended audience is younger adolescents and their parents. This highly useful and informative book makes complicated medical information accessible to teens. An index and illustrations are included.

McCoy, Kathy, and Charles Wibbelsman. **The New Teenage Body Book.** Los Angeles: Body Press, 1987. 278p.

Concerned with the overall health of teenagers, this comprehensive handbook contains sections on sexual feelings, preferences, and choices. Names and addresses of nationwide agencies that can help teenagers with health and sexual concerns are provided in the appendix. Illustrations and an index are also included. Readable and informative, this handbook is an excellent resource for teenagers.

Parrot, Andrea. **Coping with Date Rape & Acquaintance Rape.** New York: Rosen Publishing Group, 1988. 134p.

Written for male and female adolescents by one of the country's leading sex educators, this book primarily discusses the issue of date and acquaintance rape, but it also includes information about sexual decision making. A glossary, bibliography, index, and list of human resources are included.

Weston, Carol. **Girltalk about Guys.** New York: Harper & Row, 1988. 220p.

Structuring her information around real letters from teens, Weston devotes two-thirds of this book to the topics of attraction to the opposite sex, dating, and breaking up. She discusses other topics, including premarital sex, in the last part of the book. The information is solid, and the advice shows a genuine caring for teens. The author's chatty style makes the information easy to read and her advice easy to consider.

Young, Proud and Gay! Boston: Alyson, 1985. 94p.

Written specifically for gay and lesbian teenagers by gays and lesbians, this book gives information about what it means to be homosexual, coming out in school, meeting other young gays, telling your parents, gay sexuality, and finding your identity. Some ways that male and female homosexuals make love are discussed in detail. Illustrations, letters from young gays and lesbians, and annotated bibliographies enhance the text. The writing is straightforward and informative. This is an excellent resource not only for gay and lesbian readers, but for anyone wishing to broaden his or her understanding of gay sexuality.

Nonprint Materials on Sexuality

The following list represents the types of films and videocassettes available about teenage sexuality. There are, of course, many more available, but it would be impossible to list them all here. The reviewing sources for these nonprint materials included *Lander's Film Review, School Library Booklist, Media Review Digest,* and *Video Source Book.* The selections cover various viewpoints about the aspects of sexuality discussed in this chapter.

Choosing To Wait: Sex and Teenagers
Type: VHS videocassette
Length: 34 min.
Cost: Rental $75; purchase $205
Distributor: Sunburst Communications
Room RB36
101 Castleton Street
Pleasantville, NY 10570-3498
Date: 1989

This videocassette presents three couples and the different decisions they made regarding the pressures of sex. The advantages of abstinence, both for couples who are sexually active and for teens who have never had sex, are presented.

Common Sexual Problems
Type: 4 filmstrips with audiocassettes
Cost: Purchase $159
Distributor: Guidance Associates, Inc.
Communications Park, Box 3000
Mt. Kisco, NY 10549
Date: 1981

The development of sexual interest as well as the typical and temporary sexual dysfunctions of youth are the bases for this film.

Dating: Coping with the Pressures
Type: 35mm film, VHS videocassette
Length: 31 min.
Cost: Rental $75; purchase $175
Distributor: Sunburst Communications
Room RB36
101 Castleton Street
Pleasantville, NY 10570-3498
Date: 1981

Focusing on the pressures all teenagers face when their dating years begin, this videotape talks about stereotyping, sexual activity, drug use, parental attitudes, and double standards.

Deciso 3003
Type: 16mm film, VHS videocassette
Length: 8 min.
Cost: Rental $50; purchase $180 (film), $79 (video)
Distributor: Churchill Films
12210 Nebraska Avenue
Los Angeles, CA 90025
Date: 1982

In a science-fiction setting with teenagers as the main characters, students defend their right to say no.

First Things First
Type: 16mm film, VHS videocassette
Length: 30 min.
Cost: Rental $50; purchase $495 (film), $395 (video)
Distributor: Bill Wadsworth Productions
1913 W. 37th
Austin, TX 78731
Date: 1982

Girls' and boys' sexual points of view are presented through dramatizations.

The Great Chastity Experiment
Type: 16mm film, VHS videocassette
Length: 27 min.
Cost: Rental $40; purchase $490 (film), $245 (video)
Distributor: The Media Guild
11722 Sorrento Valley Road
Suite E
San Diego, CA 92121
Date: 1985

A teenage couple struggles with the decision of whether or not to become sexually active.

Hard Climb

Type:	16mm film, VHS or Beta videocassette
Length:	27 min.
Cost:	Purchase $450 (film), $400 (video)
Distributor:	Perennial Education 930 Pitner Avenue Evanston, IL 60202
Date:	1983

The patience, preparation, and mutual dependence of a climbing team are compared to the male's role in a successful sexual relationship.

He's No Hero

Type:	VHS videocassette
Length:	19 min.
Cost:	Purchase $189
Distributor:	Intermedia 1300 Dexter Avenue North Seattle, WA 98109
Date:	1989

Aimed specifically at young men, this video examines the reponsibilities of males in sexual decision making and the necessity of resisting pressures to conform to sexual stereotypes.

Homosexuality and Lesbianism: Gay or Straight, Is There a Choice?

Type:	16mm film, VHS videocassette
Length:	26 min.
Cost:	Rental $55; purchase $425 (film), $295 (video)
Distributor:	Cinema Guild 16970 Broadway, Suite 802 New York, NY 10019

A discussion on homosexuality involves high school students, a psychologist, and the president of the Community Homophile Association of Toronto.

It's O.K. To Say No Way!
Type: VHS videocassette
Length: 7 min.
Cost: Purchase $25
Distributor: YWCA of the USA
Order Department
726 Broadway
New York, NY 10003
Date: 1986

A rap music video advocates abstinence from sex.

Know How
Type: VHS videocassette
Length: 20 min.
Cost: Purchase $189
Distributor: Intermedia
1300 Dexter Avenue North
Seattle, WA 98109
Date: 1989

Comedienne Kim Coles encourages teens to postpone sexual involvement and promotes the benefits of abstinence during adolescence. She teaches teens specific skills to deal with sexual pressures.

Making Decisions about Sex
Type: 16mm film, VHS videocassette
Length: 25 min.
Cost: Rental $60; purchase $445 (film), $99 (video)
Distributor: Churchill Films
12210 Nebraska Avenue
Los Angeles, CA 90025
Date: 1981

Both sexually active and inexperienced teens talk about the seriousness of sexual commitment.

No Time Soon
Type: 16mm film, VHS videocassette
Length: 16 min.

28 SEXUALITY

Cost: Rental $75; purchase $330 (film), $300 (video)
Distributor: Select Media, Inc.
74 Varick Street
Suite 303
New York, NY 10013
Date: 1987

Two teenage friends, Vincent and Arty, discuss the general topics of sex, contraception, relationships, and teenage parenthood.

OK To Say No: The Case for Waiting
Type: VHS videocassette
Length: 30 min.
Cost: Rental $75; purchase $129
Distributor: Sunburst Communications
Room RB36
101 Castleton Street
Pleasantville, NY 10570-3498
Date: 1981

Three teenagers present the case for abstinence as an alternative to sexual intercourse. Personal choice, emotional stability, and the need to say no are stressed.

On Being Gay: A Conversation with Brian McNaught
Type: VHS or Beta videocassette
Length: 80 min.
Cost: Purchase $39.95
Distributor: TRB Productions
Focus International
P.O. Box 2362
Boston, MA 02107
Date: 1986

During an interview, gay author and lecturer Brian McNaught describes what it was like to grow up gay, recognize his homosexuality, and face family and friends about his sexual preference.

Pink Triangles: A Study of Prejudice of Lesbians and Gay Men
Type: 16mm film, VHS videocassette
Length: 34 min.

Cost: Rental $50; purchase $500 (film), $400 (video)
Distributor: Cambridge Documentary Films
P.O. Box 385
Cambridge, MA 02139
Date: 1982

Taking a look at society's attitudes toward lesbians and gay men, this video examines the nature of the discrimination they face as well as historical and contemporary patterns of racial, religious, political, and sexual persecution.

Saying "No": A Few Words to Young Women about Sex
Type: 16mm film, VHS videocassette
Length: 17 min.
Cost: Rental $35; purchase $325 (film), $275 (video)
Distributor: Perennial Education
930 Pitner Avenue
Evanston, IL 60202
Date: 1982

Young women talk about their personal decisions regarding sexuality, how they have been affected by their decisions, and how they respect themselves for having the courage and willpower to abstain from sex.

Sex and Decisions: Remember Tomorrow
Type: 16mm film, VHS videocassette
Length: 29 min.
Cost: Rental $60; purchase $495 (film), $370 (video)
Distributor: Churchill Films
12210 Nebraska Avenue
Los Angeles, CA 90025
Date: 1985

This is an appealing dramatization about the rewards of saying no to sex.

Sex and the American Teenager
Type: VHS videocassette
Length: 45 min.
Cost: Purchase $300

30 SEXUALITY

Distributor: NBC New Archives, Room 922
30 Rockefeller Plaza
New York, NY 10112
Date: 1986

Television personality Bryant Gumbel and sex advisor Dr. Ruth Westheimer are hosts of a program in which a group of sexually active teenagers discuss sexual issues.

Sex, Choices and You
Type: 16mm film, VHS videocassette
Length: 18 min.
Cost: Rental $60; purchase $395 (film), $355 (video)
Distributor: Alfred Higgins Productions, Inc.
6350 Laurel Canyon Boulevard
North Hollywood, CA 91601
Date: 1987

This film helps young people make choices regarding abstinence versus sexual activity because of the problem of AIDS and other STDs. Being responsible for oneself and one's partner is emphasized.

Sex Myths and Facts
Type: 16mm film, VHS videocassette
Length: 17 min.
Cost: Rental $60; purchase $380 (film), $340 (video)
Distributor: Alfred Higgins Productions, Inc.
6350 Laurel Canyon Boulevard
North Hollywood, CA 91601
Date: 1988

Teenagers have many misconceptions regarding sex. This highly informative film provides factual information in response to the most commonly held sexual myths.

Sexual Responsibility: A Two-Way Street
Type: VHS videocassette
Length: 30 min.
Cost: Rental $75; purchase $185

Distributor: Sunburst Communications
Room RB36
101 Castleton Street
Pleasantville, NY 10570-3498
Date: 1989

By examining the nature of responsibility in sexual relationships, this film encourages students to think about the consequences of their decisions and effective ways of dealing with their sexuality.

Sooner or Later? Issues of Teenage Sexuality
Type: VHS or Beta videocassette
Length: 43 min.
Cost: Purchase $295
Distributor: Independent Video Services
401 E. 10th Avenue, Suite 160
Eugene, OR 97401
Date: 1987

In a mock classroom, graduate-student teachers present a five-part curriculum to high school students.

Teenage Birth Control: Why Doesn't It Work?
Type: 2 filmstrips plus 2 audiocassettes, VHS videocassette; open-captioned for the hearing impaired available
Length: 25 min.
Cost: Rental $75; purchase $165 (filmstrips), $165 (video)
Distributor: Sunburst Communications
Room RB36
101 Castleton Street
Pleasantville, NY 10570-3498
Date: 1981

This video stresses that most teenage pregnancies occur because teenagers don't use birth control, even though they know about it. It also examines the emotional and psychological motivations for taking chances. A counselor leads a discussion about the safety and effectiveness of various forms of birth control.

Teenage Homosexuality
Type: 16mm film, VHS videocassette
Length: 11 min.
Cost: Rental $30; purchase $275 (film), $150 (video)
Distributor: Carousel Film and Video
260 Fifth Avenue, Room 705
New York, NY 10001
Date: 1980

Through interviews with five gay teenagers, the mother of a teenage homosexual, and a psychiatrist, this documentary provides a realistic look at the world of teenage homosexuality.

Teenage Sex: How To Say No
Type: 35mm film, VHS videocassette
Length: 43 min.
Cost: Rental $75; purchase $175
Distributor: Sunburst Communications
Room RB36
101 Castleton Street
Pleasantville, NY 10570-3498
Date: 1982

Designed for adolescents who need help in resisting the pressure for sexual activity, this video teaches how to apply assertiveness in general and specific sexual situations.

You Would If You Loved Me: Making Decisions about Sex
Type: VHS videocassette
Length: 60 min.
Cost: Purchase $209
Distributor: Guidance Associates, Inc.
Communication Park, Box 3000
Mt. Kisco, NY 10549
Date: 1988

This program is designed to help teens understand the difference between love and sex, correct sexual myths and misconceptions, examine how pressures influence responsible decision making, and encourage teens to develop their own ability to make decisions and set limits.

Organizations Concerned with Teen Sexuality

Due to the general nature of this chapter, there are no specific agencies to list for particular concerns, except in the case of homosexuality. The following groups can provide information and support for matters concerning homosexuality.

Affirmation/Gay and Lesbian Mormons
Box 46022
Los Angeles, CA 90046
(213) 255-7251
Contact: Ricky Gilbert (213) 655-3433 and Shari Glenn (213) 676-3939

Affirmation is a social support organization for gay and lesbian Mormons who are active members of the church, nonactive members, or excommunicated. The organization believes it is important that gay or lesbian individuals accept themselves within the framework of the gospel of Jesus Christ. The Los Angeles group is the umbrella organization for chapters throughout the country. The contact people will answer questions or refer you to a local chapter. You may also order informational materials from the national organization.

PUBLICATIONS: *Affinity* (newsletter) plus pamphlets about marriage, excommunication, and the scriptures and homosexuality.

Bet Mispocheh
Box 1410
Washington, DC 20013
(202) 833-1638
President of the Board of Directors: Beth Cohen

A gay and lesbian synagogue with a membership of 220 people. In addition to weekly Sabbath services, it offers social events, educational programs, and a speakers' bureau. Bet Mispocheh has been in existence for 15 years and is staffed by volunteers. It is not affiliated with a particular Jewish religious movement.

PUBLICATION: *Bet Mispocheh Newsletter* (monthly).

Beth Chayim Chadashim
6000 W. Pico Boulevard
Los Angeles, CA 90035
(213) 931-7023
Director: Rabbi Denise Eger

Beth Chayim Chadashim, a reformed synagogue with outreach for gays and lesbians, was established 18 years ago and now has almost 400 members. Its services include student outreach, social activities for all ages, and spiritual support group for members who have tested HIV-positive. Interested teens are encouraged to call for more information.
PUBLICATION: *Gvanim* (monthly).

Brethren/Mennonite Council for Lesbian and Gay Concerns
Box 24060
Washington, DC 20023
(202) 462-2595
Coordinator: Jim Sauder

BMC was founded in 1976 to provide support for Brethren and Mennonite gay, lesbian, and bisexual people and their parents, spouses, relatives, and friends; to foster dialogue between gay and nongay people in the churches; and to provide accurate information about homosexuality from the social sciences, biblical studies, and theology. The Washington, D.C., office is the BMC national headquarters and will provide information about local or regional groups affiliated with their churches.
PUBLICATION: *Dialogue* (newsletter two to three times yearly).

New Ways Ministry
4012 29th Street
Mount Rainier, MD 20712
(301) 277-5674
Director: Beverly Robinette

New Ways Ministry was founded in 1971 by Father Robert Nugent and Sister Jeannine Gramick for the purpose of educating people about sexuality. The organization's primary objective is advocacy of social justice for gay and lesbian people within the Catholic Church, but it is also concerned with homosexuals not affiliated with the church. Services include counseling, workshops, seminars, and retreats.

PUBLICATIONS: *Bondings* (quarterly newsletter), booklists, and articles.

Unitarian-Universalist Office of Lesbian and Gay Concerns
25 Beacon Street
Boston, MA 02108
(617) 742-2100
Director: The Reverend Scott D. Alexander

The Unitarian-Universalist Office of Lesbian and Gay Concerns, a nationwide clearinghouse, provides a wide range of resources and support for gay, lesbian, and bisexual religious liberals. It can provide educational materials, counseling referrals, referrals to local gay and lesbian organizations, and general support for gay, lesbian, and bisexual teenagers. The UULGC, a membership organization with many chapters around the country, can be contacted through the OLGC.

PUBLICATIONS: *UULGC World* (newsletter); "About Your Sexuality," a human sexuality curriculum that affirms gay, lesbian, and bisexual persons as normal and valuable.

Hotline

Philadelphia Gay Switchboard (215) 546-7100
Staffed from 6:00 P.M. to 11:00 P.M. daily.

Operators will answer questions and can make referrals to organizations or resources in your local area for information and services.

CHAPTER 2

Physical Development

Are you there God? It's me, Margaret. Gretchen, my friend, got her period. I'm so jealous God. I hate myself for being so jealous, but I am. I wish you'd help me just a little. Nancy's sure she's going to get it soon, too. And if I'm the last I don't know what I'll do. Oh please God. I just want to be normal.
  Judy Blume, *Are You There God? It's Me, Margaret* (New York: Bradbury Press, 1970), 100.

I woke up suddenly. It was morning. I felt wet and my pajamas were sticky. Oh God! There is something wrong with me. *Really wrong*. Dr Holland doesn't know what he's talking about! I am *so* sick. This proves it.
Wait a minute. Wait just a minute. Maybe I had a wet dream. Yeah.... I'll bet that's it. How about that?
  Judy Blume, *Then Again, Maybe I Won't* (New York: Bradbury Press, 1971), 93.

The thoughts expressed in these passages are those of 11-year-old (almost 12) Margaret Simon and 13-year-old Tony Miglione. Although these are fictitious characters, they voice feelings common among adolescents in beginning stages of sexual development.

Margaret, in *Are You There God? It's Me, Margaret*, anxiously awaits her first menstrual period because it will signify that she is a normal female. In *Then Again, Maybe I Won't,* Tony is surprised, then pleased, to have his first nocturnal emission. Although he thought at first he was sick, he knows this is not a sign of illness. But he later wonders if it is normal to have so many of these dreams. Like many adolescents, Tony and Margaret need reassurance that their development into sexually mature males and females is following a normal course. Understanding the process of physical development can provide this needed reassurance.

Male and Female Reproductive Systems

Understanding of the process of physical development entails learning about the anatomy of sexually mature males and females. It is important, and interesting, for boys and girls to know their own reproductive system and that of the opposite sex.

MALES

External genitals. The two main parts of the external male genitals, or outer sex organs, are the penis and the scrotum. The long, cylinder part of the penis is called the shaft; the top or head of the penis is called the glans. The ridge of skin around the lower part of the glans is called the corona, and the slit in the tip of the glans is the urinary opening.

If the penis is uncircumcised, there is a fold of skin, called the foreskin, covering the glans. This foreskin can be pulled down toward the shaft to expose the glans. When a penis is circumcised, the foreskin has been surgically removed.

This operation, called circumcision, is usually performed when a baby boy is a few days old. Circumcision is a religious custom among people of Jewish or Muslim faiths. For a long time, doctors encouraged parents who were not Jewish or Muslim also to circumcise their male babies because it is easier to clean the penis when the foreskin has been removed. In the last ten years, however, this practice has been questioned, and not all doctors continue to recommend routine circumcision. This is a choice parents make, and as long as the penis is cleaned properly, there is no medical reason why a male must be circumcised. The penis functions the same in either case.

When a male is sexually aroused, the shaft of the penis, which is composed of blood vessels and spongy tissue, gets longer, harder, and wider. This is called having an erection. Erections occur when the nerve center at the base of the spinal cord sends messages that cause blood to rush into the blood vessels in the penis. The muscles inside the base of the penis tighten so this extra blood can't easily drain out.

The scrotum is the sac of loose skin that hangs under the penis.

Internal genitals. Inside the scrotum are two egg-shaped organs called testicles. One testicle (usually the left) usually hangs lower than the other to avoid friction in this very sensitive part of the male body. The main function of the testicles, or testes, is to produce sperm, the tiny living cells necessary for creating a baby.

Sperm can only be produced in an environment a few degrees lower than the normal temperature of the male body. In order to maintain this exact temperature, the scrotum sometimes tightens up when the air surrounding it becomes too cold, thus drawing the testes nearer the warmth of the male's body. When the surrounding air becomes too warm, the scrotum loosens up, increasing the distance between the male's body and his testes, so they do not become too warm to produce sperm.

After sperm are produced in the tiny chambers of the testicles, they travel through the epididymis, a long, thin, tightly coiled canal that surrounds each testicle. Then they travel through the vas deferens tubes, or sperm ducts, to the seminal vesicles where they are stored. The seminal vesicles, along with the prostate gland, also produce the fluid called semen, which transports the sperm through the body.

Inside the penis is a tube called the urethra. It is connected to the bladder and carries urine from the bladder out the urinary opening. The urethra is also connected to the seminal vesicles, and carries sperm-containing semen out through the urinary opening when the male ejaculates. Ejaculation occurs when the male has been sexually aroused and semen spurts out of his erect penis. When this happens, a valve closes off the urethra so urine and semen can't mix. If the male ejaculates while he is sleeping, it is called a nocturnal emission, or a wet dream.

FEMALES

External genitals. The female's external genitals, or sex organs, are called the vulva. There are several parts to the vulva. At the top of the vulva is the mons, the fleshy mound of fat tissue that covers the pelvic bone. The two flaps or folds of skin at the bottom of the mons are called the labia majora, or outer lips. In between the two labia majora are the labia minora, or inner lips.

At the top of the area where the labia minora join together, up toward the mons, is the clitoris. Many nerve endings cluster in the clitoris, making this tiny area the most intensely sensitive place on the female body. Below the clitoris lies the urinary opening, which connects to the bladder, and beneath that is the vaginal opening. This opening may be covered or fringed by the hymen, a thin layer of perforated skin.

Some people believe that a female is not a virgin, someone who has never had sexual intercourse, if she does not have an intact hymen, but this is not true. Some girls may have been born without a hymen, and others who are virgins may have torn or stretched their hymens during vigorous physical exercise. Other females who have had sexual intercourse may still have intact hymens, although they are stretched out.

Internal genitals. Past the vaginal opening is the vagina, a canal that extends to the cervix, or neck of the uterus. The small dimple in the center of the cervix is the opening to the cervix, called the os. The uterus is the small, pear-shaped organ beyond the cervix. At the center of the uterus, or womb, is a narrow cavity. The endometrial wall, a thick, blood-rich tissue, lines the uterus.

The uterus is extremely elastic. During pregnancy, it expands to many times its original size, becoming small again after the birth of the baby. At the upper portion of the uterus, on both the right and left sides, are the Fallopian tubes. These tubes lead to the ovaries where the ova, or egg cells, are stored.

Once a month, an egg, or ovum, is released from one of the ovaries. This process is called ovulation. The egg travels through one of the Fallopian tubes into the uterus. Conception occurs if the egg is met by a sperm cell and fertilized. The fertilized egg then attaches itself to the endometrial wall of the uterus where it grows and develops into a baby. When this happens, the female is pregnant.

Each month that the female is not pregnant, the endometrial wall prepares itself for a fertilized egg by developing rich, nourishing tissue. If the egg passes in an unfertilized state, the endometrial tissue and the egg disintegrate and leave the female's body through the cervix and out the vagina as menstrual flow.

This process of ovulating and menstruating is called the menstruation cycle. Menstruating is often referred to as a female having her period. Many females experience mild or severe cramps when they menstruate. This physical discomfort is possibly caused by hormonelike substances called prostaglandins, which are produced throughout the body (Todd, 734).

Many women experience other symptoms prior to menstruation such as swelling in their breasts, weight gain, constipation, headaches, skin problems, anger, anxiety, or depression. They may also feel increased energy, sexual desire, or a sense of well-being. These symptoms are all part of the premenstrual syndrome (PMS). Some women experience a combination of positive and negative PMS symptoms, depending upon their individual body chemistry. As in the case of cramps, the exact cause for PMS has not been discovered, but the hormone progesterone may be responsible (ibid., 742).

Sexual Intercourse for Reproduction

In order for sperm to be present in the female's body, a male must ejaculate into or near her vagina. When the male inserts his penis into the female's vagina, vaginal sexual intercourse has occurred. The sperm then swim up the vaginal canal, through the os, through the cervix, through the uterus, through the Fallopian tube, and up to the ovaries. If a sperm meets a descending egg in any of these areas, conception occurs.

Just as the internal male and female sex organs prepare for reproduction by producing sperm and eggs, the external sex organs accommodate the reproduction process by facilitating the entrance of the penis into the vagina. The penis stiffens when the male has an erection, making it possible to insert it into the female's vagina and keep it there until he ejaculates. A bit of lubricating fluid is emitted from the penis to make it slide more easily into the vagina. The vagina secretes a similar fluid for the same lubricating purpose. In addition, the pleasure felt when male and female genitals rub against each other and the satisfaction of orgasm, the pleasurable release of sexual tensions, can make sexual intercourse an intensely enjoyable activity.

Sexual Development

The reproductive systems described above are those of sexually mature males and females capable of producing children. Children are born with undeveloped reproductive systems. Although eggs are present in a female's ovaries at birth, she does not ovulate until her sex organs have developed enough to support a pregnancy. Males, on the other hand, are not born with sperm in their testicles. As they mature physically, their sex organs develop so that males are capable of producing sperm and fathering children.

The time when the bodies of males and females change from those of children to those of sexually mature men and women is called puberty. Puberty takes place during the adolescent period of life. During this time, males and females experience remarkable physical and emotional changes.

These physical changes occur in predictable stages. Using the characteristics adolescent males and females commonly exhibit throughout puberty, a British doctor named J. M. Tanner has delineated five stages of sexual development (McCoy and Wibblesman, 11). Dr. Tanner's stages provide a useful framework for explaining the physical changes males and females experience and the ages at which these changes often occur.

Dr. Tanner and other experts on sexual development stress the wide range of ages considered normal within each stage. It is important to remember that although adolescents follow the same patterns of sexual development, they mature at individual rates. There is a large range for what is considered normal, and most adolescents fall within this range. The following description of the stages defined by Dr. Tanner is based on a summary of his work found in *The New Teenage Body Book* by Kathy McCoy and Charles Wibbelsman, M.D.

STAGES OF MALE DEVELOPMENT

Stage One

- Average Age: 10 Years
- Normal Age Range: 9 to 12 Years

During this stage, there are no external signs of development, but internally, testosterone, the male hormone, is becoming active. As testosterone levels increase, the boy's testicles begin to mature. Some boys have a growth spurt, or period of rapid growth, during this stage.

Stage Two

- Average Age: 12 or 13 Years
- Normal Age Range: 9 to 15 Years

During this stage, boys start to grow taller and the shape of their bodies changes as they develop new muscle tissue and add fat. They begin to look less like boys and more like young men at this stage. The areola, or circle of darker skin around the nipples on the chest, increase in size and darken a little. The testicles and scrotum begin to enlarge, but the penis does not increase in size. The skin of the scrotum reddens. Straight, fine pubic hair may begin to grow at the base of the penis.

Stage Three

- Average Age: 13 or 14 Years
- Normal Age Range: 11 to 16 Years

In the third stage, the young man continues to grow taller. His shoulders become broader, making his hips look even slimmer. His penis grows longer, but not wider. Added muscle tissues make his face and body look even more adult. The larynx enlarges during this stage, causing his voice to deepen. The testicles and scrotum continue to enlarge.

Pubic hair, which now starts to get darker and coarse, spreads along the base of the penis. Hair may also be developing around the anus, the opening at the end of the rectum. The first traces of facial hair may also appear on the upper lip during this stage.

Stage Four

- Average Age: 14 or 15 Years
- Normal Age Range: 11 to 17 Years

During this stage, the penis starts to get wider as well as longer, and the testicles and scrotum continue to grow. The pubic hair becomes more adultlike in texture, although it still covers a smaller area than it will later. Facial hair increases on the upper lip and chin. Underarm hair begins to appear. Most males have their first ejaculation during this stage, signifying that the testicles are beginning to produce sperm. The voice becomes deeper, and the skin gets oilier.

Stage Five

- Average Age: 16 Years
- Normal Age Range: 14 to 18 Years

In this stage, the male begins to look like a young adult. He has nearly reached his full height, and his physique looks like that of a mature man. He has more facial hair, and may want to begin shaving. His pubic hair has thickened and is dark and curly, like an adult's. His genitals also look like those of an adult. He may grow a bit more and add more body hair in the next few years, but the male at this point is considered sexually mature.

STAGES OF FEMALE DEVELOPMENT

Stage One

- Average Age: 9 or 10 Years
- Normal Age Range: 8 to 11 Years

In this first stage, there are no external signs of development. Internally, however, the pituitary gland stimulates the ovaries with follicle-stimulating hormone (FSH). This hormone triggers the ovaries to start producing estrogen, which is released into the bloodstream. The ovaries also begin to enlarge during this stage.

Stage Two

- Average Age: 11 or 12 Years
- Normal Age Range: 8 to 14 Years

The second stage marks the beginning of breast development. When the girl's nipples become tender and slightly raised, she is said to have breast buds. The areola, or darker skin around the nipple, also increases in size. In this stage, she experiences a growth spurt that increases her height and weight considerably. As her weight increases, her hips become broader and softly rounded with fat deposits. She will start to grow a small amount of fine, straight pubic hair during this stage.

Stage Three

- Average Age: 12 or 13 Years
- Normal Age Range: 9 to 15 Years

During the third stage, the girl grows taller and her breast growth continues. Her pubic hair, although still thin, becomes darker and coarser. Her vagina enlarges and begins to secrete a clear to whitish discharge. This fluid is part of the vagina's self-cleansing process. Some girls begin to menstruate, or get their periods, late in this third stage.

Stage Four

- Average Age: 13 or 14 Years
- Normal Age Range: 10 to 16 Years

Girls who did not begin to menstruate in Stage Three will likely do so during Stage Four. Their pubic hair, although still thin, now grows in a small triangular formation, and underarm hair begins to appear. The ovaries continue to enlarge, and some girls begin to ovulate at this point.

Stage Five

- Average Age: 15 Years
- Normal Age Range: 12 to 19 Years

In this final stage of sexual development, the female is a physical adult. She has nearly reached her full height, and her breast and pubic hair growth is completed. Her menstrual periods are well established, indicating that ovulation occurs on a regular monthly basis. She is now a young adult.

Emotions Accompanying Sexual Development

When males are able to ejaculate and females are able to ovulate, they are physically capable of producing children. Because reproduction is a biological drive, sexually mature human beings can have strong sexual urges to mate. Being physically ready for sexual intercourse, however, does not necessarily assure that young adults are emotionally ready for intense sexual activity. In contemporary American society, a teenager may be a physically mature adult, and yet still be an adolescent or child in terms of his or her emotional development. This is the dilemma confronting most teens.

In addition, many teens are anxious about their sexual development. They may be uncomfortable with the changes happening to their bodies. They may wonder if their genitals are normal, if they are or will ever be attractive to the opposite sex, if their skin will ever clear up, and so on. They may experience extreme mood shifts, feeling on top of the world one day and down in the dumps the next. Confusion, insecurity, and excitement are all emotions that accompany sexual development. Time, understanding friends and relatives, and accurate information can ease some of the pain and intensify some of the pleasure of adolescence.

REFERENCES

Bell, Ruth, et al. *Changing Bodies, Changing Lives: A Book for Teens on Sex and Relationships.* New York: Random House, 1987.

Blume, Judy. *Are You There God? It's Me, Margaret.* New York: Bradbury, 1970.

Blume, Judy. *Then Again, Maybe I Won't.* New York: Bradbury, 1971.

Eagan, Andrea Boroff. *Why Am I So Miserable If These Are the Best Years of My Life?: Everything Your Mother Never Told You about Becoming a Woman.* New York: Avon, 1988.

Hein, Karen. "Adolescence and Sexual Maturity." In *The Columbia University College of Physicians and Surgeons Complete Home Medical Guide,* ed. Donald F. Tapley, et al., 231–356. Mt. Vernon, NY: Consumers Union, 1985.

Johnson, Eric W. *Love & Sex in Plain Language.* 4th revised ed. New York: Bantam, 1988.

Madaras, Lynda, with Area Madaras. *The What's Happening to My Body? Book for Girls: A Growing Up Guide for Parents and Daughters.* New York: Newmarket Press, 1988.

Madaras, Lynda, with Dane Saavedra. *The What's Happening to My Body? Book for Boys: A Growing Up Guide for Parents and Sons.* New York: Newmarket Press, 1987.

McCoy, Kathy, and Charles Wibbelsman, M.D. *The New Teenage Body Book.* Los Angeles: Body Press, 1987.

Todd, W. Duane. "Disorders Common to Women." In *The Columbia University College of Physicians and Surgeons Complete Home Medical Guide,* ed. Donald F. Tapley, et al., 734–755. Mt. Vernon, NY: Consumers Union, 1985.

Weston, Carol. *Girltalk about Guys: Real Questions, Real Answers.* New York: Harper & Row, 1988.

Resources
for Finding Out about Physical Development

Physical Development in Fiction

The list of books in this section is brief because few books focus on a physical aspect of their characters' sexual development. Although these books contain other elements in their stories, they are examples of books that deal with specific topics concerning physical sexual development.

Blume, Judy. **Are You There God? It's Me, Margaret.** New York: Bradbury (Dell), 1970. 149p.

Margaret Simon is almost 12 years old. She is beginning to develop sexually and anxiously awaits the day when her menstrual period starts, so she will know she is normal. Throughout the book, Margaret and her friends have open discussions about bras, boys, and periods. This is one of the first novels written for young adolescents that discusses these topics.

Blume, Judy. **Then Again, Maybe I Won't.** New York: Bradbury (Dell), 1971. 164p.

Thirteen-year-old Tony Miglione has just moved to a new town. Besides making new friends and having a crush on 16-year-old Lisa, Tony also worries about his wet dreams and spontaneous erections. Embarrassed, Tony hopes no one will notice as he concentrates on developing his powers of mind over matter. This is one of the first novels written for young adolescents to discuss these topics.

Davis, Jenny. **Sex Education.** New York: Orchard Books, 1988. 150p.

Sex education is the topic for the first semester in Mrs. Fulton's ninth-grade Biology 200 class. Olivia (Livvie) Sinclair and David Kindler, project partners, study the physical aspects of sex: sexual development, the reproductive system, the stages of pregnancy. They are also assigned to look at and think about their own bodies and their sexual development.

Their project is to care about someone, and they choose to care about a young pregnant woman who lives near Livvie. They have learned enough about pregnancy to be concerned about her physical condition. They are correct in their concern, but the problem is too big for them to handle.

Nonfiction Materials on Physical Development

Most of the comprehensive books written for teens about health or sexuality have sections on the physical aspects of sexuality. The books listed here include sections that provide accurate information written in a readable fashion.

Bell, Ruth, et al. **Changing Bodies, Changing Lives: A Book for Teens on Sex and Relationships.** New York: Random House, 1987. 254p.

This comprehensive book, written specifically for teenagers, includes information on all aspects of teen sexuality and general health. Teens from across the country were consulted about its contents, and they share their views on their own sexuality and sexual experiences as a supplement to the information provided. The authors write in a straightforward manner and give a range of perspectives on each topic. Illustrations are particularly helpful in the section on male and female anatomy. This is one of the best resources available for teens.

Eagan, Andrea Boroff. **Why Am I So Miserable If These Are the Best Years of My Life?: Everything Your Mother Never Told You about Becoming a Woman.** New York: Avon, 1988. 211p.

Along with information about other topics related to general health and sexuality, Eagan includes a chapter entitled "Anatomy, Menstruation, and Getting Pregnant—What They Didn't Tell You in Biology 101." The illustrations in this section are helpful. This is a frank, honest, readable guide for young women.

Johnson, Eric W. **Love & Sex in Plain Language.** Philadelphia: Lippincott (Bantam), 1985. 207p.

Originally written in 1968, this is the fourth revision of this concise but comprehensive book. Sexual development and the male and female reproductive systems are among the topics the author discusses. Illustrations, a glossary, and an index make the information readily accessible.

Madaras, Lynda, with Area Madaras. **The What's Happening to My Body? Book for Girls: A Growing Up Guide for Parents and Daughters.** New York: Newmarket Press, 1988. 269p.

This book was written especially for younger adolescents and their parents by a leading sex educator and her teenage daughter. The primary focus is female puberty. The development of breasts, menstrual cycles, body hair, and genitals is explained in detail. Information on male puberty is also included. The frank, clear explanations and conversational writing style make information on sexual development accessible to the intended audience. Illustrations enhance the text, and an index is included.

Madaras, Lynda, with Dane Saavedra. **The What's Happening to My Body? Book for Boys: A Growing Up Guide for Parents and Sons.** New York: Newmarket Press, 1987. 251p.

Written by a leading sex educator with the assistance of a teenage boy, the book has male puberty as its primary topic. Details about the changes in physique, genitals, voice, hair, and skin are provided. There is a separate chapter on ejaculations, orgasms, erections, masturbation, and wet dreams. Information about female puberty is included. The tone is honest and conversational. The intended audience is younger adolescents and their parents. This highly useful and informative book makes complicated medical information accessible to teens. An index and illustrations are included.

McCoy, Kathy, and Charles Wibbelsman, M.D. **The New Teenage Body Book.** Los Angeles: Body Press, 1987. 278p.

Although it is concerned with the overall health of teenagers, this handbook contains sections on male and female anatomy and physical development. Names and addresses of nationwide agencies offering help for teenagers with health and sexual concerns are provided in the appendix. Illustrations and an index are also included. Readable and comprehensive, this handbook is an excellent resource for teenagers. Kathy McCoy frequently writes for teens; Charles Wibbelsman, M.D., is a specialist in adolescent medicine.

Parrot, Andrea. **Coping with Date Rape & Acquaintance Rape.** New York: Rosen Publishing Group, 1988. 134p.

Written for male and female adolescents by one of the country's leading sex educators, this book's primary focus is date and acquaintance rape. However, it is an excellent resource for information on the physical aspects of sexuality as well. It includes a glossary, bibliography, index, and list of human resources.

Nonprint Materials on Physical Development

The following videocassettes and films provide information about the male and female anatomy and puberty. The listing is by no means comprehensive, but it provides a sampling of available sources of information for teenage audiences. The reviewing sources for these nonprint materials included *Lander's Film Review, School Library Booklist, Video Source Book,* and *Media Review Digest.*

Anatomy Attitudes: Understanding Sexuality
Type: 35mm film, VHS videocassette
Length: 38 min.
Cost: Rental $75; purchase $175

Distributor: Sunburst Communications
Room RB36
101 Castleton Street
Pleasantville, NY 10570-3498
Date: 1982

This videotape stresses that healthy attitudes about sexuality will be strengthened when teens are accurately informed about anatomy and physiology. The facts about normal and abnormal development of sexual body parts are provided.

Coping with Adolescence: Understanding Puberty
Type: 4 filmstrips with 4 audiocassettes
Length: 8–12 min. per filmstrip
Cost: Purchase $119
Distributor: Learning Tree
P.O. Box 4116
Englewood, CO 80155
Date: 1981

The confusion, fears, and self-consciousness of preteens and young teens are addressed in this series on the physical and emotional changes of puberty.

Girl Stuff
Type: 16mm film, VHS videocassette
Length: 21 min.
Cost: Rental $60; purchase $440 (film), $330 (video)
Distributor: Churchill Films
12210 Nebraska Avenue
Los Angeles, CA 90025
Date: 1982

Personal appearance, hygiene, vaginal infections, and menstruation are addressed in this film about girls growing up.

Menstruation: Hormones in Harmony
Type: VHS videocassette
Length: 19 min.
Cost: Rental $35; purchase $295
Distributor: Perennial Education
930 Pitner Avenue
Evanston, IL 60202
Date: 1985

Beginning with the female anatomy, this film explains the process of menstruation.

Understanding Human Reproduction
Type: 35mm film, VHS videocassette
Length: 39 min.
Cost: Rental $55; purchase $129 (film), $145 (video)
Distributor: Sunburst Communications
Room RB36
101 Castleton Street
Pleasantville, NY 10570-3498
Date: 1984

Designed as a lead-in program to sex education, this videotape explains how conception occurs and covers the development of the fetus within the trimesters of pregnancy.

Organizations Concerned with Physical Development and Related Issues

Telephone numbers with an 800 prefix indicate there is no long-distance charge for the call.

PMS Access
Division of Medicine Pharmacy Associates
P.O. Box 9326
Madison, WI 53715
(800) 222-4PMS; in Wisconsin, (608) 833-4PMS

This organization functions as a clearinghouse for information on premenstrual syndrome (PMS). Inquiries about research and treatment are welcome.

PUBLICATION: Newsletter.

PMS Treatment Center
P.O. Box 20998
Portland, OR 97220
(503) 255-0918

This is a PMS treatment center. If you send a stamped, self-addressed envelope to the center, the staff will send you a list of other PMS treatment centers throughout the country.

Society for Adolescent Medicine
Suite 120
19401 E. 40 Highway
Independence, MO 94055
(816) 795-TEEN
Administrative Director: Edie Moore

The Society for Adolescent Medicine promotes development, synthesis, and dissemination of scientific and scholarly knowledge concerning the development of health-care needs of adolescents. This organization encourages the investigation of normal growth and development during adolescence and of those diseases that affect adolescents.

PUBLICATION: *Journal of Adolescent Health Care* (every other month).

CHAPTER 3

Contraception

"I don't want to study," he shouted.
"God, Walker." She put her hand to her throat. "You scared me."
"I got you over here on false pretenses."
"I know," she said, smiling.
"I bought prophylactics and everything."
"I bought something, too. Some kind of foam."
      Ron Koertge, *Where the Kissing Never Stops*
      (Boston: Little, Brown, 1986), 141.

"Well, we've had it. Sex, I mean. After all we've been going together since sixth grade. By the tenth—that's four years—there was nothing left to do. It sorta happened naturally. Not that I wasn't scared to death somebody would find out. I went all the way to Simmonsville to the clinic there to get a diaphragm, and I use it too. I'm faithful. So it all worked out."
      Sue Ellen Bridgers, *Permanent Connections*
      (New York: Harper & Row, 1987), 151.

"Where do you keep 'protection'?"
"Locks and alarms are against the far wall," he said, and began to walk off.
"No, I mean 'personal protection,' " I whispered.
"Have to speak up, boy."
" 'Per-son-al pro-tec-tion!' " I enunciated.

58 CONTRACEPTION

> He nodded. "Deodorant is in the cosmetics department."
>
> I shook my head. "Rubbers!" I nearly shouted. A woman shopper poked her head above the shampoos and stared at me.
>
> The pharmacist chuckled. "Come with me." I followed him down the aisle [to] ... a small display of various birth-control stuff. Rubbers. Sponges. Creams. Sprays. Goops.
>
> Larry Bograd, Travelers (New York:
Lippincott, 1986), 42.

Walker and Rachel in *Where the Kissing Never Stops* are just becoming sexually active teenagers. Leanna in *Permanent Connections* has been sexually active since she was 15. In *Travelers*, 17-year-old Jack is hoping to become sexually involved. Although their situations differ, all of these teens take precautions against pregnancy. Not only have they made conscious decisions about birth control, they know about effective contraceptive methods and how to obtain the necessary equipment. The actions of these characters reflect the behavior of real teens:

- In 1982 approximately 85 percent of sexually active teens from 15 to 19 years of age reported they had used birth control (Hayes, 46).
- Of the 9 million 15- to 19-year-olds in 1985, 2.1 million or 24 percent of the total reported using contraceptives (Pittman and Adams, 4).

Contraceptives: To Use or Not To Use

Contraception means the prevention of conception or pregnancy, so a contraceptive is a device or chemical that prevents the sperm from fertilizing the egg. Whether or not to use a contraceptive is a personal decision every sexually active teenager makes in one way or another. Although preventing pregnancy is the primary reason for sexually active teens to use contraceptives, they may be used for a variety of purposes.

Here are some common reasons for using contraceptives:

1. Birth control. Married couples use contraceptives to limit the size of their families, space the births of their children, or prevent pregnancy altogether. Contraceptives are also used outside of marriage to prevent unwanted pregnancies. Many sexually active teens use contraceptives for this purpose. Some women, even though they may not be sexually active or have sex only occasionally, routinely take birth-control pills or have an IUD inserted to protect themselves from pregnancy should they be raped.
2. Health. One form of contraception, the condom (see below), is used to protect against AIDS and other sexually transmitted diseases (see Chapter 5). Doctors may prescribe another contraceptive, the birth-control pill, to regulate a woman's hormone level and thereby control acne or lessen the intensity of cramps and other PMS symptoms.
3. Psychological freedom. Some women use contraceptives so they can say no to intercourse out of choice, not fear of pregnancy.

Here are some common reasons for not using contraceptives:

1. Sexual image. Some people feel contraceptives interfere with sexual spontaneity because they make it seem as if intercourse is a planned occurrence, not something that just happens romantically or in the passion of the moment. Some girls think the fear of pregnancy helps them avoid being promiscuous. Others fear that if they use contraceptives, their dates or boyfriends will pressure them into having intercourse because wanting to avoid pregnancy is no longer a valid excuse. Some women are too embarrassed to discuss, buy, or use contraceptives.

2. Fears. Many sexually active teens are afraid to ask their parents for contraceptives because it implies they are sexually active. They may also fear their parents will discover they are using contraceptives and are, therefore, sexually active. Some people fear side effects or long-term effects from contraceptives.
3. Lack of information. Sometimes people are unaware of effective means of contraception and/or where to get contraceptives. Others may be relying on incorrect information.
4. Inconvenience. Using contraceptives is considered too much trouble or too expensive.
5. Neglect of responsibility. When each partner thinks the other partner will or should take care of contraceptive matters, neither one may actually do it. The boy may think the girl should be responsible since she is the one who will become pregnant. The girl, on the other hand, may expect the boy to be prepared, particularly if they are not having regular sexual relations.
6. Belief systems. Some people believe all contraceptives are unnatural and interfere with the body's functioning. For others, using contraceptives goes against their religion. Catholics, for example, believe contraceptives interfere with God's will for humans to produce children.

Although the reasons for not using contraceptives are understandable, they must be weighed against the distinct possibility of unwanted pregnancy.

- "About 70 percent of women become pregnant in a year using no method of contraception" (Hein, 242).
- "Four out of every five girls who have intercourse without using birth control will become pregnant during the first year of their sexual activity" (Bell, 167).

When sexually active teens seriously consider the consequences of having sexual intercourse without contraceptives and learn the facts about birth control, concerns and fears about contraceptives often diminish. Teens with philosophical or religious convictions that oppose the use of contraceptives often feel a particular obligation to avoid artificial means of contraception. In any case, the decision to become sexually active demands a decision about contraceptive use. As the saying goes, "not to decide is to decide"; in the case of birth control, failing to make a conscious decision about contraceptive use means that it would be okay if the girl became pregnant.

If pregnancy is unwanted, the girl and her partner must decide what method of birth control is acceptable. Having a broad knowledge of birth-control methods provides more versatility in case a backup method is needed or if a temporary method is required before arrangements for a regular method are made.

Birth-Control Methods

There are three ways to prevent conception: abstinence, nonprescription methods, and prescription methods. Each method has advantages, disadvantages, and specific information related to its use. Methods vary in ease of use and effectiveness. The statistics for effectiveness rates are constantly being updated as more information becomes available. Whenever possible, the following numbers reflect recent data that relate specifically to teenagers using birth control.

ABSTINENCE

Complete abstinence. Refraining from sexual intercourse at all times is called complete abstinence. The biggest advantage of complete abstinence is that it is 100 percent effective in preventing pregnancy if the penis never enters or ejaculates near the vagina.

Its disadvantage is that sometimes couples who refrain from sexual intercourse engage in other sexual activities that could lead to pregnancy. Because sperm survive in a warm environment, they can remain alive outside the vagina. Therefore, even if the boy ejaculates near the girl's vagina rather than in it, the live sperm could later enter the vagina and cause pregnancy. However, there are other ways for couples to express love safely and satisfy each other sexually, making it possible for some teens to maintain their convictions about abstinence. (See Chapter 1.)

Periodic abstinence or natural birth control. Natural birth control requires abstinence from vaginal sexual intercourse during the girl's fertile period. It relies on understanding when ovulation occurs (that is, when the ovary produces an egg) and avoiding sexual intercourse before, during, and after ovulation, a time span of about 10 to 12 days.

There are three ways to determine when ovulation will most likely occur. The first is the rhythm or calendar method. This method involves calculating the number of days from the first day of one period to the first day of the next. Ovulation usually occurs around the middle of the cycle. Therefore, in the case of a girl who has a 28-day cycle, ovulation would occur on the fourteenth, fifteenth, or sixteenth day of her cycle, counting from the first day of the girl's last period. She should definitely not have intercourse on these days.

In addition, sperm can live in the girl's body for up to six days, so she should not have intercourse for six days prior to ovulation. Therefore, her fertile period begins on the eighth day. In addition, the egg usually stays in the girl's body from two to four days, so another four days must be added to the abstinence period, making it extend to the twentieth day. Thus the "safe" time to have intercourse for a girl with a regular 28-day cycle would the first seven and the last seven days of her menstrual cycle—and the first three to seven days will probably be her period.

The advantage of using the rhythm method is that it is in keeping with religious or philosophical teachings that object to mechanical or chemical interference with reproduction. Religious organizations advocating its use usually provide information and counseling for married women using the rhythm method.

The biggest disadvantage to the rhythm method is that it does not effectively prevent pregnancy.

- The rhythm method is 72 percent effective against pregnancy when used by women under 20 years of age (Jones and Forrest, 106).
- Out of 100 sexually active teenage females who use the rhythm method, about 28 will become pregnant (ibid.).

The rhythm method has a higher percentage of pregnancies than any of the other birth-control methods discussed in this chapter. One reason for this high rate of failure is that very few girls under the age of 22 have regular menstrual cycles, so it is difficult to predict when ovulation will occur. Stress, travel, sickness, weight gain, or weight loss can make a period come early or late. In addition, ovulation can sometimes occur at unusual times, like during the girl's period.

It is also possible that a hardy sperm or two may survive in the girl's cervix longer than the usual two to four days. Therefore, the egg may still meet a sperm even though the girl does not engage in sexual intercourse during her estimated fertile period. Another disadvantage is that the rhythm method provides no protection against sexually transmitted diseases. (see Chapter 5).

The second way to determine when ovulation occurs is by the mucus method. This method involves daily examination of the different types of mucus secreted from the cervix.

When the girl is not fertile, there is either very little mucus around her cervix or it is thick and white. Four to six days before ovulation, the mucus becomes thinner and clearer. Right before ovulation, the mucus is stringy and elastic, resembling raw egg white. Sperm thrive in this mucus, and it enables them to swim up the Fallopian tubes where they meet the egg. After ovulation, the mucus disappears again or returns to a thick, white state.

The girl must use her finger to remove a bit of mucus from her cervix each day to check the state of the mucus. During the time the mucus is clear, stringy, and elastic, and four days after it disappears (indicating ovulation is over), girls practicing the mucus method must abstain from sexual intercourse. This is usually eight to ten days out of the girl's menstrual cycle.

The advantages of the mucus method are the same as those of the rhythm method. Its biggest disadvantage is that its failure rate is about the same as that of the rhythm method because it is often difficult to read the mucus signs. Semen remaining in the vagina from intercourse may look and feel like mucus. Special training and supervision are necessary to use this method well. It also requires regularity; forgetting to check the mucus for one day may mean missing a sign that the girl is fertile.

The third method for determining ovulation is the temperature method. This form of natural birth control involves taking the girl's temperature with a special basal thermometer each morning before she gets out of bed and recording it on a special chart. Twenty-four to thirty-six hours before ovulation, the girl's temperature usually drops slightly. It then rises after ovulation. Accurately recording the girl's daily temperature, therefore, helps determine when she ovulates and can become pregnant.

The advantage of the temperature method is the same as that of the mucus and calendar methods—none of them requires physical or chemical barriers to interrupt the union of the egg and the sperm.

The disadvantage of the temperature method is that it has a high failure rate similar to that of the rhythm method. This high rate of pregnancy probably occurs because the temperature method only indicates that ovulation will occur in a day or two and when ovulation has occurred. Since the fertile period starts up to six days before ovulation, the information the temperature method provides can come too late. It also requires the girl to keep careful records. Illness, of course, can throw these records off.

Simultaneous use of all three of these methods requiring periodic abstinence is the most effective way to achieve natural birth control, but it requires that the girl be exceptionally aware of her own body and highly disciplined about keeping records.

NONPRESCRIPTION CONTRACEPTIVES

Many types of contraceptives can be purchased at grocery stores, drugstores, and family-planning centers without a doctor's prescription. This means that contraceptives are available to everyone, even though some teens find it embarrassing to buy them. Understanding what they want before going to purchase contraceptives may ease this awkwardness. The prices quoted here are those of the retail stores, but they are often lower at clinics. Some clinics even provide free contraception.

Condoms. A condom (rubber, safe, prophylactic, skin, sheath, bag, Trojan, Sheik, protection) is a thin, latex rubber sheath (a tube that is closed at one end) that fits over the boy's erect penis just before intercourse. When the boy ejaculates, the condom catches the semen he emits so it does not come in contact with the girl's body.

- Condoms are about 86 percent effective in preventing pregnancy among females under the age of 20 (ibid.).

A box of three condoms costs between $1.00 and $1.50. They are usually found on the shelves in the pharmacy section, but some restrooms have vending machines where they may be purchased. They come in all colors, and one size fits everyone.

Prelubricated condoms are coated with a wetting agent that makes them easier to put on, but also makes it more likely that they may slip off during intercourse. K-Y jelly and saliva are effective lubricants for nonlubricated condoms, but using petroleum jelly or any substance containing oil will weaken the rubber.

There are no health risks involved in using the condom and no side effects either. They should be stored away from heat, including body heat, so carrying them in a pocket or wallet is not a good idea.

To use a condom, tear open the tinfoil packet, take out the rolled-up condom, and unroll it onto the erect penis. This must be done before intercourse, even before the boy's penis comes close to the girl's vagina, because even a few drops of the lubricating fluid from the boy's penis can contain enough sperm to make the girl pregnant. When placing the condom on the penis, leave at least one-half inch of slack at the tip to collect the semen so it will not leak out the other end. Some condoms have a special tip for this purpose.

It is important to remove the penis from the vagina as soon after ejaculation as possible, before the penis returns to normal size, so the condom does not slip off. It is crucial to hold the end of the condom so all the semen stays in the condom. Then remove the condom and throw it away. Drying the penis before it comes near the girl's vagina again is essential because even a few drops of semen can cause pregnancy.

The condom's advantages include being safe, effective, and easy to get. Since condoms are the only effective form of birth control that boys can use, they give a male the opportunity to be sexually responsible, even if the girl has bought them and hands them to him at the crucial moment. Condoms that contain the spermicide (sperm-killing) nonoxynol-9 (n-9) are the most effective, and they also protect against AIDS and some other sexually transmitted diseases (see Chapter 5). There are no health risks, short- or long-term, for condom users.

One disadvantage of the condom is that some males complain that unlubricated condoms interfere with their sexual satisfaction. However, the lubricated kinds or the kinds made from animal membrane do not seem to present this problem and feel like bare skin. Other couples complain that using condoms interferes with the spontaneity of lovemaking because they cannot be put on ahead of time. Couples who make putting on a condom part of the process of intercourse don't seem to find this too much of an inconvenience.

A bigger disadvantage is that, when used alone, condoms are only 86 percent effective. The 14 percent chance of pregnancy comes from the fact that it only takes one sperm to fertilize an egg. Therefore, one drop of semen leaking from the condom or a bit of lubricant dripping from the penis prior to putting on the condom can cause pregnancy.

Foam. Contraceptive foam is a spermicide that contains a chemical that kills the sperm in the boy's semen. About 15 to 20 minutes before intercourse, the foam is inserted into the girl's vagina with an applicator much like a tampon. The foam spreads out evenly in the vagina where it blocks the sperm from entering the cervix and remains until it is absorbed. This characteristic makes foam more effective than other spermicides, like jellies and creams.

- Used alone, contraceptive vaginal foam is about 82 percent effective in preventing pregnancy in women of all ages (Hein, 242).

An aerosol can of contraceptive foam that contains about 20 applications costs about $3. A plastic applicator tube may come with the container, or may be purchased separately. Foam also comes in individual doses prepackaged in disposable applicators. A box of six individual applications costs about $3. Although the individual applications are more expensive, they are more convenient and can be carried in a purse like tampons.

Foam can be purchased at supermarkets, drugstores, and family-planning centers. It is usually found on the shelf with other birth-control and feminine-hygiene products.

There are no health risks involved with using foam, but sometimes a boy will find that a particular brand irritates his penis, and occasionally a girl will use a brand that irritates her vagina. An aerosol container of foam is effective up to a year and a half after it is manufactured, and should be stored away from heat.

To use foam, shake the can well, place the plastic applicator over the top of the can and press down. The foam will squirt out into the applicator. When the applicator is full, remove it from the can. Then gently push the applicator into the vagina, pointing it toward the cervix. (It's probably easiest to do this while lying down.) To release the foam, push the plunger all the way to the top of the applicator. To be safe, use two applicators of foam.

Although foam can be inserted right before the penis enters the vagina, it can also be inserted up to half an hour before intercourse. This application must be repeated before each intercourse. Inserting an additional dose of foam after intercourse is a good idea. In order to give the spermicide time to work effectively, the girl should not plan to swim, douche, or bathe for about six hours following intercourse. (That's how long it takes to kill all the sperm.) It is also a good idea to have an extra can of foam available since it is impossible to tell when the can is getting close to empty.

The advantages of foam include being inexpensive, easy to use, and easy to get. In addition, some types of foam can protect against sexually transmitted diseases (see Chapter 5). Girls who have sex irregularly and do not want to use a daily form of birth control, like the pill or the IUD, often find foam a convenient contraceptive method.

Foam does have its disadvantages. Some people think it is messy, both when inserting it and after intercourse, particularly if more than one application is used. Others, as mentioned, find particular brands irritating and, therefore, uncomfortable.

But the biggest disadvantage of foam is the relatively low level of protection it provides against pregnancy. Not making the foam cover the cervix, not using enough, inserting the foam too early, or being too active after inserting it can cause the foam to fail. If the girl swims or bathes less than six hours after intercourse, the foam will wash away and fail to kill all the sperm.

Foam and condom. Although the biggest disadvantage of both condoms and foam is their ineffectiveness, when used in combination, they provide "almost perfect protection against pregnancy" (Eagan, 111). If a bit of semen should spill from the condom, the spermicide in the foam will prevent pregnancy; if the foam is improperly applied, the condom will prevent most of the sperm from entering the vagina.

This backup system has a 98 percent effectiveness rate (Bell, 174). It also enables both partners to participate actively in the process of birth control.

In addition, using a condom eliminates the irritation some boys experience from some brands of foam. But most importantly, using the foam/condom combination provides the best protection known against the AIDS virus (except for abstinence) and other sexually transmitted diseases (Eagan, 111). (See Chapter 5.)

Jellies and creams. Spermicidal jellies and creams are substances inserted into the vagina to prevent the sperm from entering the cervix. They come in tubes and are applied before intercourse. A small tube that contains enough for about 10 applications costs between $2 and $3. A large tube containing enough cream or jelly for about 20 applications costs about $5. They can be purchased at grocery stores, drugstores, or family-planning centers. They are usually placed among feminine-hygiene and birth-control products.

Although jellies and creams are applied the same way foam is, they are considered less effective because they do not spread out like foam does, and therefore do not protect the cervix as well.

- Couples using only contraceptive jelly or cream have a 34 percent chance of becoming pregnant (Jones and Forrest, 106).

The advantages of creams and jellies are that they are easy to use and easy to get. They also are good protection against sexually transmitted diseases (see Chapter 5). The biggest advantage of creams and jellies is that when used with a diaphragm (as described below), they provide excellent protection against both pregnancy and sexually transmitted diseases.

Their biggest disadvantage is their low level of effectiveness in preventing pregnancy when used alone. They are also messier to use than foam, and may irritate the penis or vagina.

Suppositories. Contraceptive suppositories are large tablets that are inserted into the vagina by hand or with an applicator fifteen minutes to one hour before intercourse. The movement during intercourse causes them to melt and mix with body fluids. They come in boxes of 10 to 16 tablets per box and can be bought in drugstores and some supermarkets for $5 to $7 per box. Although they are easy to purchase and use, like other spermicides except foam, they are not very effective in preventing pregnancy.

- Vaginal contraceptive suppositories are only 66 percent effective in preventing teenagers from becoming pregnant (ibid.).

They are not even as effective as foam because they do not spread the spermicide they contain evenly throughout the vagina; the cervix is therefore inadequately protected.

Sponge. Made out of plastic foam and filled with the spermicide nonoxynol-9, the sponge measures about one-and-three-quarters inches in diameter. It is donut-shaped with an indentation (instead of a hole) in its center, which fits over the cervix and blocks sperm from entering. A polyester loop or ribbon attached to the outside of the plastic enables it to be removed easily.

The sponge is 80 to 85 percent effective in preventing pregnancy (Eagan, 110). It can be purchased at supermarkets, drugstores, and family-planning clinics for about $1.

To use the sponge, wet and insert it into the vagina before intercourse, making sure it covers the cervix. It can be left in place for up to 24 hours and is designed to protect against pregnancy no matter how many times sexual intercourse occurs within that time period. However, it must be left in place for 6 hours after intercourse is completed, so there is actually only an 18-hour period in which intercourse may take place. The sponge should not be used during the girl's period, and it should never be left in place for more than 24 hours.

The biggest disadvantage of the sponge is its low protection rate. It can also irritate the cervix and may cause foul odors. Sometimes the ribbon breaks when the sponge is being removed, and the girl must have the sponge removed at a clinic or emergency room.

The advantages of the sponge are its availability and its convenience over an extended time period. It also protects against sexually transmitted diseases. Using the sponge with a condom can greatly increase its effectiveness against pregnancy.

PRESCRIPTION CONTRACEPTIVES

Because the third type of contraceptives requires a prescription, the girl must be examined by a doctor before she can use any of them. Many girls are afraid of this examination and avoid it, thereby limiting their birth-control options. Knowing what to expect in a gynecological examination can make it less intimidating.

Gynecological examination. A girl considering using a prescription contraceptive must first make an appointment for a gynecological examination. These examinations vary in cost from $30 to $40. Some girls feel comfortable discussing this matter with their parents and decide to go to the family doctor or their mother's gynecologist (a doctor who specializes in female health concerns).

Other girls choose to visit family-planning clinics, women's clinics, free clinics, or doctors recommended by friends. Names, addresses, and telephone numbers of local clinics can be found in the Yellow Pages under Clinics. One advantage to going to a clinic is that they frequently deal with teenage girls and understand their concerns.

Many girls shop around before making the appointment. They call clinics or doctors' offices and ask the cost of the exam, how often they deal with teenagers, whether parental permission is needed before seeing a doctor, if any of the doctors are women (if this is important to the girl), where they are located, and how to go about making an appointment. They note the manner of the person answering these questions because this indicates whether the people there will be respectful and friendly to teens.

Some girls find that taking a parent or friend along with them to the appointment may make them feel more at ease and helps pass the time since there is usually a lot of waiting involved. While she is waiting for the doctor, the girl will be asked to provide a complete medical history. The medical history concerns the girl's present and past health and the health of her family (another good reason for bringing a parent along).

Before seeing the doctor, a nurse or an assistant will ask the girl to go into the bathroom and supply a urine sample. Then she will be directed to an examining room where she will undress (in private) and slip on a hospital gown. A nurse or assistant will come in and take her blood pressure, measure her height and weight, and take a blood sample. If the doctor is a man, a female nurse or assistant will probably stay with the girl during the examination. She can request this if it does not happen automatically.

When the doctor arrives, he or she will conduct a general check of the girl's eyes, ears, nose, throat, teeth, skin, glands, heart, lungs, pulse, and reflexes. Then the girl will be asked to lie on her back on the examining table and put her hands behind her head. The doctor will gently feel around the girl's breasts to check for lumps. Then he or she will look at and feel the patient's outer genitals. Because the girl's reproductive organs are inside her body, the doctor must look and feel inside her vagina. This is called a pelvic exam.

During the pelvic exam, the girl positions herself at the end of the examining table with her legs spread apart, her knees bent, and her feet in special metal supports called stirrups. A sheet is placed across her knees. The doctor inserts two gloved fingers into the girl's vagina and checks the uterus for abnormalities or pregnancy by holding the cervix and using his or her other hand to gently press the lower abdomen from the outside. The doctor also feels the Fallopian tubes and ovaries, checking for cysts or abnormalities.

It is also necessary for the doctor to look inside the girl's vagina to check for infections or pregnancy. To do this he or she uses an instrument called a speculum to hold open the walls of the vagina so the doctor can see the vaginal walls and cervix. Inserting the speculum and opening it up to separate the vaginal walls can be uncomfortable for the girl, particularly if she is tense. Concentrating on relaxing can be helpful during the speculum exam.

While the speculum is in place, the doctor will carefully scrape some cell tissue from the cervix with a long swab or flat wooden stick. These cells will be used for a test called a Pap smear which helps identify cancer of the uterus. After the speculum is removed, the doctor may want to check the girl's rectum for lumps and swelling. To do this, he or she will gently insert one finger into the girl's anus. This is called a rectal exam.

Throughout the gynecological exam, the doctor should explain what he or she is doing and why. The doctor will ask the girl questions about her periods and answer any question she may have, either before, during, or after the exam. Her doctor is the patient's best source for information about what types of contraceptives would be best for her, and the matter should be thoroughly discussed before she makes her final decision and the doctor gives her the prescription.

It is essential that the girl understand how to use the contraceptive she chooses before she leaves the doctor's office. However, knowing as much as possible about the various contraceptives before her discussion with the doctor can eliminate confusion and expedite her decision. A gynecological exam is necessary for the diaphragm, the pill, and the IUD.

Diaphragm. The diaphragm is a soft, flexible rubber cup that fits over the girl's cervix and prevents the sperm from entering the cervix. Diaphragms come in various sizes and need to be personally fitted. They are used with a contraceptive jelly or cream that functions as a lubricant and a spermicide. A doctor's prescription is required for the diaphragm, but not for the contraceptive jelly, which was described above.

The diaphragm generally costs about $15, not including the doctor's exam. The diaphragm will probably come with some contraceptive cream or jelly at first, but more must be purchased at the drugstore or supermarket when that supply is used up.

- Used with the jelly, the diaphragm is 97 percent effective against pregnancy (Bell, 179) and has "no adverse medical consequences" (Hein, 242).

The diaphragm must, however, be properly in place whenever sexual intercourse occurs. The cream or jelly offers double protection against a tiny sperm slipping past the rim of the cup should it not fit properly. It also protects against sexually transmitted diseases (see Chapter 5).

To use the diaphragm, the girl coats the inside of the cup with about a tablespoon of jelly, folds the diaphragm in half, and gently pushes it into her vagina until it covers her cervix and presses against her pelvic bone. It is a good idea to practice doing this ahead of time to make sure it is done properly. The diaphragm can be inserted while the girl is sitting, standing, or lying down. Once it is in place, neither the girl nor the boy should be able to feel it.

It can be inserted up to two hours before intercourse, but the closer to the time of intercourse, the better. An additional dose of cream or jelly must be inserted with an applicator if the couple decides to have intercourse more than once. The diaphragm must remain in place for eight hours after intercourse. The girl should not swim, bathe, or douche during these eight hours or the spermicidal jelly will be washed away and pregnancy may occur.

The diaphragm is removed by inserting a finger between its rim and the cervix to gently break the suction and slide it out. It should be washed after each use and dusted with cornstarch or potato flour (not talc, which may contain bits of asbestos), and stored away from heat because heat can dry out the rubber. A diaphragm usually lasts about two years. It can be checked for tiny holes by holding it up to the light.

Used with spermicidal cream or jelly, the diaphragm has the advantage of being a safe, easy to use, highly successful birth-control device. Also, the diaphragm is only used when a couple wants to have intercourse and, therefore, does not affect the girl's body chemistry throughout the rest of her menstrual cycle. The contraceptive jelly used with it can also protect against sexually transmitted diseases.

Its disadvantage is that it must be inserted every time the couple has intercourse. Sometimes a girl might not have it when she needs it or she may forget to use it. Some girls find it messy to insert the cream and others feel embarrassed about putting a diaphragm on in front of the boy or excusing themselves to do so.

Intrauterine device (IUD). The IUD is a small plastic or plastic and metal device that the doctor inserts into the girl's uterus to prevent contraception. IUDs come in a variety of shapes—loops, coils, rings, and shields—and sizes. Although no one knows exactly how the IUD works, it is an effective form of birth control.

- The IUD is 94 to 96 percent effective in preventing pregnancy among females of all ages (ibid.).

The IUD itself costs around $200 and there is an additional charge of about $100 for insertion. Girls wishing to use the IUD have it implanted during their periods by a doctor. This process can be uncomfortable and may result in some initial cramping, but after the IUD is in place, all the girl needs to do to be protected against pregnancy is to make sure the IUD's strings are hanging into the opening of her cervix. She should check this daily.

Although the IUD has the advantages of convenience and a very high success rate for preventing pregnancy, it has many disadvantages. IUDs can cause excessive bleeding, which can lead to anemia. They provide no protection against sexually transmitted diseases, and they increase the chances of germs getting into the uterus and Fallopian tubes. They also increase the risk of developing pelvic inflammatory disease (PID), which may make it impossible for the girl ever to become pregnant.

In addition, an IUD may poke a hole in the uterus. It may become embedded in the uterus or misplaced and have to be surgically removed. An IUD can come out by accident without the girl's knowing it, like during her period, and pregnancy can occur. There have recently been many lawsuits against the makers of IUDs, and doctors usually do not advise teenagers to use this method of birth control.

The pill. The birth-control pill contains artificial hormones that interrupt the normal production of eggs so the girl no longer ovulates. Because she produces no eggs, the girl cannot become pregnant. The pill is a highly effective contraceptive.

- The pill, if used properly, is 98 percent effective against pregnancy among females of all ages (ibid.).

The hormones in the pill also change the lining of the uterus in such a way that even if an egg were produced and fertilized, it could not be implanted in the uterus, making pregnancy impossible in this way as well.

A girl using the birth-control pill must have a doctor's prescription for the pill best suited to her system. Some pills have lower doses of the hormone estrogen, for example. Pills usually come in packets containing 28 pills, one for each day of the girl's menstrual cycle, 7 of which are iron pills the girl takes during her period. Each of the other 21 pills contains enough artificial hormones to make the girl's body cease to ovulate (because it "thinks" it's pregnant).

If the girl takes her pill at the same time each day, she maintains an even hormonal level and the chances of pregnancy are slim. If she forgets to take a pill on schedule, she must take it as soon as she remembers and continue to take the next one on schedule. If she forgets and skips a whole day, she must take two the next day. Missing two pills means the girl should continue to take the pills, but she should use another form of birth control, like foam and condoms, that month to be safe from pregnancy.

Also, if a girl is taking antibiotics, she should use an additional form of birth control because these medications may interfere with the pill's effectiveness. It costs between $6 and $8 a month to take birth-control pills.

The advantages of the pill are that it is effective and does not interfere with spontaneous sexual intercourse. It can also reduce premenstrual tension and menstrual cramps and clear up acne.

There are, however, side effects from taking the pill. Some girls experience symptoms of pregnancy—weight gain, nausea, tender breasts, headaches—when they begin taking the pill, but these usually disappear with time or with a change in the type of pill taken. A smaller number of girls experience severe headaches, leg cramps, and depression.

The pill does not protect against sexually transmitted diseases and seems to weaken the body's resistance to viral infections. Its long-term effects are still largely unknown as it has only been on the market for about 20 years.

However, "serious health risks from oral contraceptive use are lower for young women under age 20 than for other age groups" (Tyrer, 92). All things considered, the majority of sexually active teenagers wishing to avoid pregnancy choose birth-control pills (ibid., 93).

With so much information to consider, deciding which type of birth-control method to use can seem like an overwhelming task. But the importance of the task makes it worth serious consideration. When choosing a method of birth control, sexually active teens may find it helpful to answer the following questions:

How important is it to me to be protected?

What would the consequences be if the girl became pregnant?

Can I rely totally on my partner to take care of birth control?

What can I do to prevent pregnancy?

Can I reasonably expect myself to take the responsibility of using the contraceptive regularly and correctly?

Do I understand any side effects or health risks that might be involved with a particular form of birth control?

Will this method protect against sexually transmitted diseases?

Fallacies about Birth Control

There is a lot of misinformation floating around about ways to prevent pregnancy. Here are some common misconceptions about conception:

- You can't get pregnant if you have intercourse while standing up.
- The girl can't get pregnant during her period.
- You can use plastic wrap or a baggie instead of a condom.
- The girl can't get pregnant if the boy withdraws his penis before he ejaculates.
- Douching (with anything) will prevent pregnancy.
- The girl can't get pregnant the first time she has sexual intercourse.
- Girls under 15 can't get pregnant.
- You have to be 15 years old to buy contraceptives.
- If the girl urinates right after intercourse, she can't get pregnant.

Conclusion

The wide variety of birth-control methods available makes it possible to select a contraceptive that satisfactorily meets individual needs and preferences. As the regularity of intercourse and the consequences of intercourse change throughout a person's life, he or she may wish to use different forms of birth control. Making informed decisions about birth control is the first step that sexually active teenagers take toward being sexually responsible. The second step is using the method of choice every time they engage in sexual intercourse.

REFERENCES

Bell, Ruth, et al. *Changing Bodies, Changing Lives: A Book for Teens on Sex and Relationships.* New York: Random House, 1987.

Bograd, Larry. *Travelers.* New York: Lippincott, 1986.

Bridgers, Sue Ellen. *Permanent Connections.* New York: Harper & Row, 1987.

Eagan, Andrea Boroff. *Why Am I So Miserable If These Are the Best Years of My Life?* New York: Avon, 1988.

Hayes, Cheryl D., ed. *Risking the Future: Adolescent Sexuality, Pregnancy, and Childbearing.* Vol. 1. Washington, DC: National Academy Press, 1987.

Hein, Karen. "Adolescence and Sexual Maturity." In *The Columbia University College of Physicians and Surgeons Complete Home Medical Guide,* ed. Donald F. Tapley, et al., 231–356. Mt. Vernon, NY: Consumers Union, 1985.

Jones, Elise, and Jacqueline Forrest. "Contraceptive Failure in the United States," *Family Planning Perspectives* 21, no.3 (May/June 1989): 106.

Koertge, Ron. *Where the Kissing Never Stops.* Boston: Little, Brown, 1986.

Pittman, Karen, and Gina Adams. *An Advocate's Guide to Numbers.* Washington, DC: Children's Defense Fund, 1988.

Tyrer, Louise. "Teenagers and OCs." In *Managing Contraceptive Pill Patients* by Richard P. Dickey, M.D., Ph.D. 5th ed. New Orleans: Creative Infomatics, 1987. 92–93.

Resources
for Finding Out about Contraception

Contraception in Fiction

In most of the young-adult novels listed below, some form of contraception is used by teenage characters. Although using birth control is usually just a part of these stories, this aspect is highlighted here.

Adler, C. S. **Binding Ties.** New York: Delacorte (Dell), 1985. 183p.
Even in the midst of their passionate lovemaking, Anne and Kyle remember to use condoms. Anne visits Planned Parenthood, but the book does not describe the visit in detail.

Betancourt, Jeanne. **Sweet Sixteen and Never...** New York: Bantam, 1987. 136p.
Julie has just turned 16 when she starts dating Sam Stewart. Sam is much more sexually experienced than Julie, who is a virgin, but he takes it very slowly with her. When Julie decides it's time she consider birth control, she visits Planned Parenthood. Julie's mother discovers Julie's pills and confronts her.

Blume, Judy. **Forever.** Scarsdale, NY: Bradbury (Pocket Books), 1975. 220p.
Katherine and Michael start going together during the second half of their senior year in high school. When they start to become sexually active, Katherine insists Michael

wear a condom, which he does. Later she goes to Planned Parenthood, where she has a gynecological exam and gets the pill.

Bograd, Larry. **Travelers.** New York: Lippincott, 1986. 184p.
Jack Karlstad agrees to drive with his wealthy friend Wendell to California for a long weekend. Wendell's main objective is to have a good time and lose his virginity. Before they leave, he sends Jack to buy condoms so they will be prepared. Jack accomplishes this task, even though he encounters his English teacher while making his purchase. As it turns out, the boys don't need to use the condoms after all.

Bridgers, Sue Ellen. **Permanent Connections.** New York: Harper and Row (Harper Keypoint), 1987. 264p.
While caring for his uncle in a small mountain village in North Carolina, Rob meets Ellery. They make love spontaneously one afternoon, but argue afterward when Rob wants to do it again. Rob thinks having protection is all they need to worry about, but Ellery wants to talk about their feelings. Ellery talks to her cousin, Leanna, and discovers she and her boyfriend, Travis, are sexually active. Leanna uses a diaphragm.

Koertge, Ron. **The Arizona Kid.** Boston: Little, Brown, 1988. 228p.
Billy leaves his family and friends in Bradyville, Missouri, and spends the summer in Arizona. He falls in love with Cara Mae, and they share their first sexual experience. Thanks to his uncle's foresight, Billy is prepared for the situation with condoms.

Koertge, Ron. **Where the Kissing Never Stops.** Boston: Little, Brown (Dell), 1986. 224p.
In an open, honest relationship, Rachael and Walker share their feelings about their own bodies and the use of contraception. Although the couple does not use a birth-control method the first time they have intercourse, they do after that. One scene describes how they use foam and condoms.

Levy, Marilyn. **Putting Heather Together Again.** New York: Ballantine (Fawcett Juniper), 1989. 136p.

When 17-year-old Heather discloses that she has been a victim of date rape, her stepmother takes her to a rape crisis center to talk to a counselor. To make sure she is not injured, Heather has her first gynecological exam. As her doctor describes the procedures, the reader learns about this type of medical examination.

Mazer, Harry. **I Love You, Stupid.** New York: Crowell (Flare), 1981. 185p.

While making plans to lose their virginity together, Marcus and Wendy discuss the possibility of Wendy taking's the pill or having an IUD inserted. They decide that Marcus should buy condoms, which they use.

Strasser, Todd. **A Very Touchy Subject.** New York: Delacorte (Dell), 1985. 181p.

Scott Tauscher, 17, lives next door to Paula Finkel who is a sexually active 15-year-old. She has an older boyfriend who sneaks out of her window every morning at 8:15 A.M. Paula tells Scott she lets her boyfriend use her sexually because she needs to feel close to someone. Paula uses birth-control pills, but when her alcoholic mother discovers them she physically abuses Paula.

Zindel, Bonnie. **Hollywood Dream Machine.** New York: Viking (Bantam), 1984. 179p.

Seventeen-year-old Gabrielle Fuller spends the summer with her best friend, Buffy, whose family has moved from New York to California. Buffy has changed. She has a boyfriend whom her parents allow to share her room on weekends. Buffy was on the pill, but forgot to take it for four days and became pregnant.

Nonfiction Materials on Contraception

Although most of the following sources contain information about more than birth control, their sections on contraceptives provide informative and accessible material for teens to consider. These sources vary in the amount of detail they provide.

BOOKS

Bell, Ruth, et al. **Changing Bodies, Changing Lives: A Book for Teens on Sex and Relationships.** New York: Random House, 1987. 254p.

This comprehensive book includes information on all aspects of teen sexuality and general health. It was written specifically for teenagers. The section on birth control explains how different types of contraceptives work, their rates of effectiveness, and their advantages and disadvantages. Teens from across the country share their views on and experiences with various birth-control methods.

The authors write in a straightforward manner and provide many useful details. The photographs and illustrations are particularly helpful in the birth-control section. This is one of the best resources available for teens.

Eagan, Andrea Boroff. **Why Am I So Miserable If These Are the Best Years of My Life?: Everything Your Mother Never Told You about Becoming a Woman.** New York: Avon, 1988. 211p.

Along with other topics associated with sexuality and general health, Eagan discusses birth control. She describes the various methods and how to use them, with diagrams, and discusses the advantages and disadvantages involved. She clearly states her views about the lack of research on the pill and the IUD and the dangerous side effects of each.

Johnson, Eric W. **Love & Sex in Plain Language.** Philadelphia: Lippincott (Bantam), 1985. 207p.

Originally written in 1968, this comprehensive but concise book is in its fourth revision. The author covers basic information about sexuality and sex. In a chapter on contraception, he explains the various types of birth control, how to use them, and their rates of effectiveness. This book is readable and the illustrations, glossary, and index make the information readily accessible.

Madaras, Lynda, with Area Madaras. **The What's Happening to My Body? Book for Girls: A Growing Up Guide for Parents and Daughters.** New York: Newmarket, 1988. 269p.

This book was written especially for younger adolescents and their parents by a sex educator and her teenage daughter. Although the primary focus is female puberty, the authors also include information on methods, safety, and effectiveness of birth control. Madaras believes it is important to provide young teens with information about contraceptives before they need it. The frank, clear explanations and conversational writing style make this information accessible, and illustrations enhance the text. An index is included.

Madaras, Lynda, with Dane Saavedra. **The What's Happening to My Body? Book for Boys: A Growing Up Guide for Parents and Sons.** New York, Newmarket, 1987. 251p.

Written by a sex educator with the assistance of a teenage boy, the primary topic of this book is male puberty. The section on birth control explains methods of contraception and the effectiveness and safety associated with each. This book's intended audience is younger adolescents and their parents. Madaras believes it is important for boys to have birth-control information before they actually need it. The illustrations, index, and conversational tone make this a very readable and informative book.

Weston, Carol. **Girltalk about Guys.** New York: Harper & Row, 1988. 220p.

Weston devotes two-thirds of this book to the topics of attraction to the opposite sex, dating, and breaking up. She includes a brief section on birth control in which she discusses talking about birth control with parents and provides information about several types of contraceptives. The author's chatty style makes the information easy to read.

ARTICLE

"Can You Rely on Condoms?" *Consumer Reports* (March 1989): 135–141.

The research staff of *Consumer Reports* tested various brands of condoms for their effectiveness against breakage. They also surveyed 3,300 readers about their use of condoms and knowledge about AIDS. Detailed reports of this research are given in this article.

Nonprint Materials on Contraception

This list is a sampling of the types of films, videocassettes, and filmstrips available about contraception. Reviewing sources included *Lander's Film Review, Video Source Book, School Library Booklist, Media Review Digest,* and Planned Parenthood video selections.

The Birth Control Movie
Type: 16mm film, VHS videocassette
Length: 24 min.
Cost: Rental $45; purchase $425 (film), $375 (video)
Distributor: Perennial Education
930 Pitner Avenue
Evanston, IL 60202
Date: 1981

This informative yet lighthearted film portrays the facts about contraception to younger audiences.

Condom Sense
Type: 16mm film, VHS videocassette
Length: 25 min.
Cost: Purchase $450 (film), $400 (video)
Distributor: Perennial Education
930 Pitner Avenue
Evanston, IL 60202
Date: 1981

A bold and humorous program concentrating on male responsibility and caring in a sexual relationship.

Condom-eze
Type:	VHS videocassette
Length:	5 min.
Cost:	Purchase $95
Distributor:	Intermedia
	1300 Dexter North
	Seattle, WA 98109
Date:	1988

Without showing human anatomy, this short film demonstrates the proper way to use a condom.

Contraceptive Choices
Type:	VHS or Beta videocassette
Length:	16 min.
Cost:	Rental $50; purchase $250
Distributor:	Milner-Fenwick, Inc.
	2125 Greenspring Drive
	Timonium, MD 21093
Date:	1985

The various types of contraceptives available and the effectiveness of each type are discussed.

Contraceptive Update
Type:	VHS videocassette
Length:	30 min.
Distributor:	Health Communications Network
	Division of Television Services
	Medical University of South Carolina
	171 Ashley Avenue
	Charleston, SC 29425
Date:	1980

This program provides information on IUDs and oral contraceptives.

Hope Is Not a Method III
Type:	16mm film, VHS videocassette
Length:	22 min.

Cost: Rental $45; purchase $450 (film), $400 (video)
Distributor: Perennial Education, Inc.
930 Pitner Avenue
Evanston, IL 60202
Date: 1984

This program covers all the birth-control methods presently available. The discussion of each method explains how the method works, how it should be used, its effectiveness rate, and any drawbacks. Available in Spanish.

It's O.K. To Say No Way!
Type: VHS videocassette
Length: 7 min.
Cost: Purchase $25
Distributor: YWCA of the USA
Order Department
726 Broadway
New York, NY 10003
Date: 1986

This rap music video advocates abstinence from sex.

No Time Soon
Type: 16mm film, VHS videocassette
Length: 16 min.
Cost: Rental $75; purchase $330 (film), $275 (video)
Distributor: Select Media, Inc.
74 Varick Street
Suite 303
New York, NY 10013
Date: 1987

Topics of sex, contraception, relationships, and teenage parenthood are discussed via the friendship of teenagers Vincent and Arty.

Pelvic and Breast Examination
Type: 16mm film, VHS videocassette
Length: 12 min.
Cost: Rental $35; purchase $235 (film), $185 (video)
Distributor: Perennial Education, Inc.
930 Pitner Avenue
Evanston, IL 60202

Date: 1975

This program shows the cervix, instruments used for a pelvic examination, and how a pap smear and a gonorrhea culture are taken. It demonstrates how relatively painless these tests are and encourages women to self-examine their breasts regularly and visit their doctor at least annually.

Sexual Abstinence: The Right Choice?
Type: VHS videocassette
Length: 30 min.
Cost: Purchase $185
Distributor: Guidance Associates, Inc.
Communications Park, Box 3000
Mt. Kisco, NY 10549
Date: 1989

This program stresses that abstinence from sexual intercourse is the only 100-percent effective protection against unwanted pregnancy and sexually transmitted diseases, such as AIDS.

Teenage Birth Control: Why Doesn't It Work?
Type: 2 filmstrips with audiocassettes, VHS videocassette
Length: 25 min.
Cost: Rental $75; purchase $129 (filmstrips), $165 (video)
Distributor: Sunburst Communications
Room RB36
101 Castleton Street
Pleasantville, NY 10570-3498
Date: 1981

Even though teenagers know about birth control, they must use it or pregnancy will occur. There are only two choices in responsible sex: abstinence or birth control. The six most often used reasons for failing to use birth control are cited and the inherent fallacies of each are discussed.

The Teenage Pregnancy Experience
Type: 16mm film, VHS videocassette
Length: 26 min.

Cost: Rental $48; purchase $370 (film), $315 (video)
Distributor: Parenting Pictures
121 NW Crystal Street
Crystal River, FL 32629
Date: 1981

Pregnant teenagers and high school–age parents examine their reasons for not using birth control and discuss their unwanted pregnancies.

Organizations Concerned with Contraception

There are many organizations that provide birth-control information and services for teens. The best source in most areas is the local Yellow Pages of your telephone directory. Look under the headings of Birth Control, Contraception, Adolescent Clinics, Family Planning, or Planned Parenthood. Other sources of information may be counseling agencies, school counselors, public libraries, and community service hotlines.

Planned Parenthood Federation of America, Inc.
810 Seventh Avenue
New York, NY 10019
(212) 541-7800
President: Faye Wattleton

Planned Parenthood Federation of America, Inc., is the nation's oldest and largest voluntary family-planning organization, tracing its origins to the first birth-control clinic in America founded in 1916 by Margaret Sanger. Planned Parenthood is dedicated to the principle that every individual has the fundamental right to choose when or whether to have children. Services provided by local chapters include gynecological examinations, birth-control counseling, contraception for males and females, female sterilization, and vasectomies. Consult your local phone book for the Planned Parenthood clinic in your area.

PUBLICATIONS: Pamphlets on a variety of reproductive health-care topics.

Society for Adolescent Medicine
Suite 120
19401 E. 40 Highway
Independence, MO 94055
(816) 795-TEEN
Administrative Director: Edie Moore

This organization is concerned with improving the quality of health care for adolescents. If you send a stamped, self-addressed no. 10 envelope to the above address, the staff will mail you a list of adolescent clinics in your area where you can obtain services including gynecological exams and birth-control counseling.

PUBLICATION: *Journal of Adolescent Health Care* (every other month).

CHAPTER 4

Teenage Pregnancy

"I'm three and a half months pregnant," Lauren said, looking straight at each of her parents in turn.

"Lauren!" her mother screamed. She sat without moving, as if she were carved out of stone.

"Pregnant? What do you mean pregnant?" her father said, looking at her, puzzled.

"Oh, Dad," Lauren said, starting to cry.

Harriett Luger, *Lauren* (New York: Viking, 1979), 42.

Lauren is 17 years old. She and Donnie are in love and have been going together for five months. Although Lauren suspects something is wrong when she misses her periods, she rationalizes, saying she is always irregular and it will probably come tomorrow. When she finally tells Donnie, he encourages her to get an abortion. Lauren's and Donnie's parents also want her to have an abortion and argue over who should pay for it.

Angry and confused, Lauren runs away from home and is taken in by two single mothers struggling to live on welfare. Lauren is very unhappy and attempts suicide. After an agonizing month away from home, she returns home and reconciles with Donnie and her parents. At first, Lauren hopes Donnie will marry her, but he has college plans and is not ready for marriage. Lauren then hopes her parents will support her while she lives at home and raises her child, but her parents' unhappy marriage makes this plan impossible. What can she do?

Although Lauren is a character from a novel, this is a question that many real teenagers must face. As the following statistics indicate, teenage pregnancy continues to be a widespread occurrence in the United States.

- Over 1 million teenagers become pregnant each year (U.S. House of Representatives, 6).
- One teenage girl in ten will become pregnant each year (Mecklenburg and Thompson, 24).
- Four out of ten girls currently 15 years old will become pregnant sometime during their teens (ibid.).

Pregnancy occurs for teenage women in all racial or socioeconomic groups in American society. The general figures given above can be broken down further, showing a bit more precisely the ages and backgrounds these 1 million pregnant teens represent.

- 54,530 girls under the age of 15 became pregnant in 1981 (Henshaw, 95).
- 549,380 15-to-17-year-olds were pregnant in 1981 (ibid.).
- 739,290 18-to-19-year-olds were pregnant in 1981 (ibid.).
- Of the 1.1 million teen pregnancies that occurred in 1978, black teenagers were more likely than whites to have unplanned pregnancies and births; 82 percent of pregnancies and 70 percent of births among blacks were unintended, compared to 71 percent of pregnancies and 49 percent of births among whites (Guttmacher Institute, 20).

Recognizing Pregnancy

SIGNS OF PREGNANCY

Lauren, the fictitious character referred to earlier, experienced some classic signs of pregnancy, but tried to deny them. Denial is a common reaction to an unintended pregnancy, but the following signs should alert sexually active teenagers to the possibility of pregnancy.

1. Skipping a menstrual period is the most obvious indication of pregnancy, but many teens have irregular periods or do not keep exact records. They are uncertain when their periods are due, and may not suspect pregnancy until they are more than a month along. In addition, some women mistake the spotting that can occur during pregnancy for a period and believe they are not pregnant.
2. Gaining weight.
3. A thickening at the waist that makes it difficult to fasten jeans that recently fit.
4. Nausea, often called morning sickness, queasiness, or vomiting can occur any time of day, particularly during the first trimester (first three months) of pregnancy. Some pregnant women cannot tolerate the smell of cigarette smoke or other strong odors. Others find the sight of food makes them nauseous.
5. Tender, swollen breasts, particularly if this condition does not precede a menstrual period.
6. The need to urinate more frequently than usual.
7. Feeling more tired than usual.

Any of these occurrences may signal pregnancy.

PREGNANCY TESTS

A teen who suspects pregnancy should have a pregnancy test as soon as possible. A pelvic exam (see Chapter 3) and a doctor's checkup should immediately follow a positive pregnancy test.

Urine tests. Urine tests can detect the presence of a special pregnancy hormone called HCG. Urine tests can be conducted in a lab or clinic or at home, using a home pregnancy-test kit. Home kits can be purchased for about $10 to $15 and used two weeks after a missed period.

A positive result in a urine test means the woman is pregnant; a negative reading, however, does not always mean she is not. The test should be repeated in about a week if it is negative and the woman still has not menstruated.

Blood tests. A blood test can also detect the presence of HCG. Blood tests can be obtained at clinics and doctors' offices for around $15 to $25. They are 99 percent accurate and identify pregnancy ten days after conception, even before a missed period (Witt and Michael, 36).

Emotional Responses to Pregnancy

Discovering an unintended pregnancy can be a very shocking experience, and coping with it can be traumatic. Many pregnant teens respond to their pregnancies much as Lauren did. A typical response of a pregnant teen is denial, thinking, "It couldn't happen to me." Then she may use a home pregnancy test or visit a clinic to confirm her suspicions.

Anger and confusion are typical reactions at this point. She may be angry at herself for letting it happen, at the guy for getting her into the situation, and at her friends who remain carefree.

She is confused about what to do. How can she tell her parents, the baby's father, her friends? Should she have an abortion, get married, ask her parents or the baby's grandparents to support her and the baby? She may feel depressed, as do many pregnant teens, and consider or attempt suicide at some point.

Finding someone with whom she can discuss her feelings is essential for a pregnant teen. Some teens are close to their parents or other family members and can discuss the situation with them. Parents are usually upset initially, but many turn out to be very understanding and supportive. Some girls turn to the baby's father or other friends. Others choose to share their problems with school nurses, guidance counselors, teachers, ministers, rabbis, priests, social workers, or psychologists.

With a supportive person to help her understand her feelings and examine the choices she has to make, a pregnant teen will be better able to sort out her emotions and make decisions that are best for the baby and everyone else involved. The decisions are difficult, but once they have been made, many pregnant teens feel calmer and ready to focus on what they must do.

Choices

Teenage pregnancy is not a new phenomenon, but the options available to today's teens are somewhat different from those of 30 years ago. At that time, when a teenager got pregnant, she and the boy either married quickly and had a "premature" baby, or the girl went to live in a maternity home where she privately waited out the pregnancy and then gave the child up for adoption. Abortions did occur, but they were illegal and either performed by a black-market doctor or someone medically unskilled. Rarely did an unmarried teen mother keep her child unless it was adopted by her parents and raised as her sister or brother.

But times have changed. Although the basic choices—abortion, marriage, or adoption—are still the same, the circumstances surrounding each of these is different.

The first choice a pregnant teen must make is whether she will terminate the pregnancy by having an abortion or continue the pregnancy to full term and deliver the child.

ABORTION

Many teens are not prepared for motherhood. They may not feel mature or responsible enough to raise a child. They may feel deep anger and resentment at being pregnant. They may have plans to finish high school and go to college. They may have grown up in fatherless homes and not want to make another child do the same.

While these may be the same reasons teens give for releasing their babies for adoption, many girls feel they could not give a child up after carrying it for nine months and so choose to terminate the pregnancy. As the following figures reveal, abortion is an option selected by many pregnant teenagers.

- 400,000 teens are estimated to have abortions each year (U.S. House of Representatives, ix).
- About 41 percent of teenagers who are pregnant have abortions (Pittman and Adams, 27).
- Two-thirds of the pregnant girls younger than 15 do not carry their pregnancies to full term (ibid., 11).
- In general, the higher a teenager's socioeconomic status, the more likely she is to terminate pregnancy by abortion (Guttmacher Institute, 52).

It is only in the last 15 or so years that teens have had the legal option of abortion. In the 1973 case of *Roe v. Wade*, the U.S. Supreme Court ruled that the decision to have an abortion during the first trimester was up to the woman and her doctor. However, states may regulate abortion during the riskier second three months for the protection of the mother's health. Individual states may regulate and even forbid abortion entirely after six months, except in cases where the mother's life and health are in danger.

The 1976 Supreme Court decision in the case of *Planned Parenthood v. Danforth* stated that a mature minor needs no one's permission to obtain an abortion. However, more recent decisions have ruled that a minor may need to have a judge determine whether she is mature. Some states require that parents be notified, but the choice to have an abortion is legally their daughter's.

A teenage woman's decision regarding abortion usually involves her belief about when life begins. Some people believe life begins when the egg is fertilized. These people are generally opposed to all abortions. Other people believe life doesn't begin until around the fifth month of pregnancy and feel it is all right to have an abortion during the first three months of pregnancy. Others justify abortions during the first six months because they believe a fetus does not become a human life until it can survive outside the uterus, which is at about 25 weeks.

Even though the decision is legally hers, a teen considering an abortion often finds it helpful to discuss her views about when life begins and her plans for her own life with her parents and/or some type of counselor before making the final decision. Although the decision should not be made hastily, the type of abortion she would have depends on how far along she is in the pregnancy.

The medical definition of an abortion is "the ending of a pregnancy before the fetus has developed enough to live outside the uterus" (Richards and Willis, 57). A pregnancy that ends by itself is called a spontaneous abortion or miscarriage. Estimates indicate that around 10 to 15 percent of teen pregnancies end in miscarriage (Pittman and Adams, 10).

When a doctor terminates the pregnancy, it is called an induced abortion, commonly referred to as an abortion. Abortions are medical procedures performed in clinics or doctors' offices and they require appointments. Some clinics offer pre- and postabortion counseling, which many teens find helpful.

First trimester abortion. The type of abortion done in the first 12 weeks of pregnancy is a surgical procedure called a vacuum aspiration. The procedure itself takes from two to seven minutes, but the whole process—admission, counseling, tests, and recovery—can take from four to six hours in a clinic or doctor's office, making an overnight stay in the hospital unnecessary. A vacuum aspiration costs from $150 to $300.

To perform this type of abortion, the doctor inserts a plastic tube into the cervix, which has been numbed with a painkiller and held open with metal rods. The tube, which the doctor rotates inside the uterus, is attached to a sucking machine called a vacuum aspirator. The suction from the machine breaks up the fetal tissue and pulls it from the uterus. Vacuum aspiration is the safest, least painful, most effective, and most commonly used early method of abortion (Richards and Willis, 60).

Dilation and curettage (D & C) is a surgical method of abortion that can also be performed during the first trimester, most often from the eighth to the twelfth week of pregnancy. It does not require an overnight stay in the hospital and costs about $200. After the patient is given a general anesthestic, the cervix is dilated and tissue is scraped from the uterus with a curette, a spoon-shaped metal object. Although this is a safe procedure, it involves a greater risk of infection and more discomfort, bleeding, and clotting than the vacuum method of abortion (ibid., 61).

Second trimester abortion. A D & C may be performed during the second trimester, but it involves an overnight hospital stay and, therefore, costs about $380. As with all inpatient procedures, it will most likely require parental consent.

Dilation and evacuation (D & E) is another second-trimester surgical procedure. It sometimes requires an overnight stay in the hospital and costs between $400 and $650. It is usually done between the thirteenth and sixteenth weeks of pregnancy, but can be performed safely up to the eighteenth and possibly even twenty-fourth week. To dilate the cervix more fully in this more advanced stage of pregnancy, a small stick of compressed seaweed is inserted the day before the surgery. The surgery itself takes 10 to 20 minutes and is a combination of scraping and suction.

Between the sixteenth and twenty-fourth weeks, a hypertonic saline abortion (salt solution) or a prostaglandin (synthetic hormone) abortion can be performed. This type of abortion is really a medically induced miscarriage. It must be done in a hospital and requires parental consent for a young teen. It may require a hospital stay of up to three nights and costs between $650 and $800 or even more.

The patient is given a local anesthetic and then the salt or hormone solution is injected directly through the abdomen into the amniotic sac. The solution causes the uterus to contract, as it would in childbirth, and a miscarriage occurs. The fetus comes out between six hours and two days after the injection. The placenta usually follows the fetus, but if it does not, it must be scraped out. Although this method is usually successful, occasionally the contractions fail to push the fetus out and it must be removed surgically.

Both these types of abortion are riskier than other methods and have the disadvantage that the fetus may be born alive and survive for a few minutes. Occasionally the fetus lives longer, but often has brain damage. However, the risk of giving birth to a live fetus can be avoided by having the abortion before the twentieth rather than the twenty-fourth week of pregnancy (ibid., 63–64).

Delayed abortions also have severe health risks for the mother. According to the Alan Guttmacher Institute, "the risk of death and major complications from abortion rises with every week the procedure is delayed after the eighth week" (55). This fact is especially pertinent to teenagers because teens are more likely than women in their twenties to obtain abortions during the later weeks of pregnancy, and "the younger the teenager, the more likely she is to have a delayed abortion" (ibid.).

HAVING THE BABY

Health concerns. If a teen decides not to have an abortion, she has chosen to have the baby. For every two girls who conceive, one will choose to give birth (Pittman and Adams, 11). It is important that the girl who opts to give birth receives prenatal (before birth) care as soon as possible to avoid health problems for herself and her baby. Many pregnant teens encounter health problems because their "bodies are still growing and their endocrine systems are inadequately developed" (Oettinger, 17). The serious health hazards that threaten pregnant teens are well documented:

- The risk of maternal death (death as a result of pregnancy or childbirth) is 60 percent higher for girls under the age of 15 than it is for older girls (ibid.).
- The risk of maternal death for girls from 16 to 19 is 13 percent higher than for girls who wait until they are in their 20s to bear children (ibid.).
- Mothers under 19 years of age are more likely to miscarry, hemorrhage, or suffer toxemia in serious forms involving high blood pressure, seizures, and death; the risk of each of these is higher for girls under 15 (ibid.).
- The health of pregnant teens under 15 is at greatest risk (U.S. House of Representatives, 1).

- Even if they deliver safely, teenage mothers are still apt to suffer postnatal anemia (Oettinger, 17).
- Growth of the adolescent mother may be stunted since the potential for optimum height is not reached until four to five years after first menses (ibid., 17–18).

Babies of teen mothers are also high risks for health problems. One major problem is that many babies born to teenage mothers have low birth weights. This is a serious concern because "low birth weight is a major cause of infant mortality, as well as a host of serious childhood illnesses, birth injuries and neurological defects, including mental retardation" (Guttmacher Institute, 29). The following statistics show the magnitude of the low-birth-weight problem:

- Out of all low-birth-weight births, 20 percent of these babies are born to teens (Pittman and Adams, 4).
- Of all the babies born to teens in 1983, almost 10 percent had low birth weights (U.S. House of Representatives, xiii).
- The younger the teen, the greater the chance her child will have a low birth weight (Pittman and Adams, 17).
- Infants born to adolescents have significantly higher rates of low birth weight and infant mortality than do other infants (U.S. House of Representatives, xiii).

Prenatal care. Because health risks are high for both mother and baby, proper prenatal care is essential. Since teenagers are still developing physically, pregnant teens need extra nutritional care. Unfortunately, many teenagers have poor eating habits, which can lead to health and developmental problems in their babies.

The fact is that the baby will take what nourishment it needs first, at the undernourished mother's expense, leaving her body nutritionally deficient. Therefore, as soon as possible, pregnant teens should visit a doctor's office or clinic. There the doctor or nurse will regularly check on the health of the teen and the development of her baby. She will be advised to exercise daily, rest when she is tired, and eat a nutritionally balanced diet, such as the following, which is recommended by the National Dairy Council. A pregnant teenager's daily diet should include:

1. Four or more servings of dairy products, skim milk, ice cream, yogurt, cottage cheese, and cheese
2. Three servings of meat, fish, eggs, or an equivalent protein source such as cheese, cottage cheese, dried beans, or peanut butter
3. Four servings of fruits and vegetables, including at least one green leafy vegetable
4. Four servings of a whole grain or cereal, like bread, oatmeal, grits, or pasta

In addition, it is important *not* to:

1. Take drugs of any kind, including aspirin, alcohol, caffeine, or medications not prescribed by a doctor who is aware of the pregnancy
2. Smoke or be around people who are smoking cigarettes
3. Have X-rays taken
4. Eat junk food

Eating properly improves the chances that the baby and the mother will be healthy, not only during the pregnancy, but in the future as well. Unfortunately, many pregnant teens do not receive the best prenatal care, and they and their babies suffer the consequences. Although 18-to-19-year-olds are slightly more likely to have better health care and better pregnancy outcomes than younger teens, women aged 20 and over generally receive better health care than do teenagers (U.S. House of Representatives, 1). Generally speaking, the younger the teen, the less likely she is to have adequate prenatal care (Pittman and Adams, 17).

ADOPTION

Sometimes teens who carry a pregnancy to full term and deliver their babies choose to relinquish their babies for adoption. Some of these are girls who might have wanted an abortion but waited too long, leaving themselves no choice but to have the baby. Others have moral or religious convictions that prevent them from having an abortion, but do not feel prepared for parenthood. And some initially planned to marry, then changed their minds, and decided against single parenthood. Because they understand that "an adoptable baby is at a premium and will always be placed in a good home" (Oettinger, 80), these teens choose to let their babies be adopted.

After deciding on relinquishment (giving the baby up for adoption), the teen still has many decisions to make. She may want to leave home and live with friends or relatives until she delivers the baby. Many girls feel more comfortable getting away from the immediate situation if their family and friends disagree with the decision to relinquish or cannot provide the emotional support they need. Others may not want to be around people they knew before the pregnancy and elect to live in a maternity home until the baby is born.

However, because teen pregnancy does not carry the stigma it once did, this option is less frequently chosen these days, and many of the Florence Crittenton and Salvation Army maternity homes have been closed or converted to parent-education centers for teenagers. In fact, many girls who elect to relinquish remain at home and attend their own schools or special programs for teen parents until they deliver their babies.

Types of adoption. Another decision that teens intending to relinquish must make involves the type of adoption they wish to have. Sometimes a family adoption, which means having the child adopted by a member of the mother's or father's family, seems to be a good idea. Family adoptions are legal in all states and can be easily arranged without an agency. However, it may be difficult for the biological mother to pretend to be the child's sister or cousin and not have a say in how the baby is raised (Richards and Willis, 138).

Another type of adoption that also does not involve using an adoption agency is a private adoption. Private adoptions are arranged between the natural parents and the adoptive parents with the approval of the courts. Many laws governing private adoptions have been made "to keep people from buying and selling children or just giving them away . . ." (ibid., 137).

Many attorneys and counselors advise against private adoptions, other than family adoptions, because it is so difficult to screen adoptive parents and match them to the babies. Private adoptions can involve many legal problems. Dealing with a reputable agency will ensure the proper legal process is followed.

Using an adoption agency means the teen selects an agency whose function is to screen prospective adoptive parents and effectively match them with babies for adoption. These agencies are either private or public institutions. Some private agencies have specific church or religious affiliations. Other private agencies and all public agencies are not religiously affiliated.

Agencies often provide counseling to the teen to help her decide if she really wants to relinquish the child and to help her cope with the emotions she is experiencing. After agencies have screened potential adoptive parents, they may give the natural mother several case histories to review. This gives her a chance to indicate what religious, professional, or cultural background she prefers the adoptive parents to have.

Of course, she will not know their names, and they will not know hers. The baby's birth certificate can even be changed so it does not indicate that the child was adopted. Some biological mothers choose to include a letter to the adoptive parents or the baby explaining why the child was released for adoption. This helps the natural mother know her decision will be understood by the child and his or her new parents.

Although most states do not keep track of the age of an adopted baby's natural mother, the following statistics from a national survey show that relatively few teens choose the option of adoption.

- In 1982, 3 percent of the infants born to unmarried teenagers were placed for adoption (U.S. House of Representatives, 19).

- In 1982, 7 percent of white unmarried teens gave their babies up for adoption (ibid.).
- In 1982, the rate for black babies released for adoption was less than 1 percent (ibid.).

MARRIAGE

Teens who do not relinquish their babies for adoption choose to raise the child themselves. Some teen mothers choose to raise the child on their own and others marry. Marriage is an option for couples who feel they have a stable, long-term relationship and who feel ready to accept the responsibilities of raising a child together. In the past more teens chose this option than do today.

- In 1960, more than one-half the girls who conceived premaritally and continued their pregnancies were married; however, in 1980, only one-third of teen women with premaritally conceived babies chose marriage (Pittman and Adams, 15).
- About 8 percent of pregnant teens under the age of 15 choose marriage (ibid., 17).
- About 30 percent of pregnant teens between the ages of 15 and 17 choose marriage (ibid.).
- For pregnant teens between the ages of 18 and 19, about 49 percent choose marriage (ibid.).

The decision to marry is a difficult one, and it sometimes requires parental consent. Unless the baby has already been born and the mother has been legally declared an emancipated minor, girls under the age of 18 must have parental consent before they can obtain a marriage license. The age may be higher or lower in some states.

As with any other important decision involving teen pregnancy, it is helpful to discuss the situation with parents, friends, and others who will listen and counsel the young couple. Matters such as money, education, jobs, and expectations of one another and of the marriage need careful consideration before the decision to marry is made.

LIVING TOGETHER

Some couples are not sure they want to marry and decide to live together instead. They reason that it will be easier to avoid legal entanglements should they decide to separate.

Witt and Michael caution that there are "problems associated with living together, however, especially for the young woman and her child" (88). Generally speaking, the woman has no legal rights to any material goods accumulated during the time she and her boyfriend are living together. She and the baby are not covered by any life and/or health insurance her boyfriend may have from his job.

If he is injured, becomes seriously ill, or dies, she has no legal say in what happens to him. She will not automatically receive his life insurance or his Social Security benefits should he die. The same is true for him if the situation were reversed. Like any of the other decisions involving pregnancy, living together needs to be thoughtfully considered before a couple chooses it.

SINGLE PARENTING

Many teens decide to keep their babies and raise them on their own. In fact, "more than half of teens who give birth are single when their child is born" (Pittman and Adams, 10). If they are young teens, they may continue to live with their own parents, receiving financial and emotional support from them. Often these girls feel they could not make it on their own and are relieved when their parents offer help.

Others feel that living with parents does not allow them enough independence. They consider help and advice from their parents to be interference and want to live on their own. Public assistance programs, like Aid to Families with Dependent Children, are available to eligible single mothers.

Other Concerns

SCHOOLING

Pregnancy can be disruptive to a teen's schooling. All the emotional trauma often makes it difficult for her to concentrate on her studies. In addition, she may miss school because she does not feel well or must keep appointments during school hours. Although schools cannot legally forbid pregnant girls to attend public schools, some teens find it impossible to meet the requirements of a regular junior high or high school program.

Many school districts have special school programs tailored to meet the needs of the pregnant teen. Some girls feel much more comfortable attending schools where everyone is in the same boat and the staff is specially trained to understand the needs of pregnant students. Other girls choose to take the high school equivalency test and are thus able to graduate. Unfortunately, as the following figures reveal, many pregnant teens drop out of school and do not ever finish.

- Pregnancy causes high school women to drop out of school more than any other factor (Richards and Willis, 151).
- Of girls who become pregnant as high school sophomores, 51 percent drop out of school before graduation (Pittman and Adams, 17).
- Teenagers who are under the age of 18 when they have their first child are more likely to drop out of school than those who delay childbearing (Hayes, 126).

POVERTY

The chances that a pregnant teenager will live much of her life in poverty are high because "poverty and poor employment opportunities are closely associated with nonmarital childbearing" (ibid., 119).

- 54 percent of families headed by single females are poor (ibid.).
- 73 percent of unmarried teens go on welfare within four years after the birth of their first child (Pittman and Adams, 27).
- In 1975, half of the over $9 billion spent on public welfare in the Aid to Families with Dependent Children program went to families begun when the mother was a teenager (Oettinger, 17).

REPEAT PREGNANCIES

Many teens become pregnant not only once but several times during their teenage years, as the following statistics show:

- Three-fifths of all teen pregnancies are second pregnancies (Witt and Michael, 153).
- About 43 percent of teen mothers have a second child within three years (Pittman and Adams, 27).
- Some 25 percent of those whose first pregnancy ended in abortion have a repeat pregnancy within two years (Hayes, 203).

While having one child as a teen negatively affects a young woman's educational and economic opportunities, a second child severely compounds the problems wrought by teen pregnancy.

FATHERS' ROLES AND RIGHTS

Much of the focus on teenage pregnancy centers on expectant teenage mothers, but of course the fathers must also be considered. Many boys experience feelings similar to the girls' feelings when they learn they have fathered a child. They often feel angry, confused, and depressed. They may also feel helpless and unnecessary.

Some boys want to assume the responsibilities of fatherhood, but lack the financial ability and emotional maturity to do so. Some want nothing to do with the situation. Others remain involved and help the girl as much as possible. Whatever their individual reactions and decisions, most young men want to understand their legal rights and responsibilities.

In terms of an abortion, the decision is made by the mother with the advice of her doctor. While some pregnant teens may want to consider the child's father before deciding, they are not legally required to. The father is not legally required to help with the cost of the abortion, although many men offer to pay or share the expense.

In the case of adoption most states do not require the consent of an unmarried father before the child is released, but he does have the right to be notified if his identity is known. If the father is opposed to the adoption, he may be given permission to raise the child himself.

Of course, the father has a say in whether he marries the mother or not.

Conclusion

Teenage pregnancy will change the lives of more than one million adolescents in the United States each year. Abortion, delivery, marriage, single parenting, and adoption become serious considerations for these teens. There are no easy answers.

Abortion may be physically and mentally risky, but so may the health of a teen carrying her child to term. In addition, the health of babies born to teenagers is frequently at risk. Teens who elect to keep their babies are more likely to drop out of school, have difficulty finding employment, have a repeat teen pregnancy, and live in poverty than their peers. The problems of pregnant teens are shared by all members of society.

REFERENCES

Alan Guttmacher Institute. Teenage Pregnancy: *The Problem That Hasn't Gone Away*. New York: Alan Guttmacher Institute, 1981.

Hayes, Cheryl D., ed. *Risking the Future: Adolescent Sexuality, Pregnancy, and Childbearing.* Vol. 1. Washington, DC: National Academy Press, 1987.

Henshaw, S. K. "A Portrait of American Women Who Obtain Abortions," *Family Planning Perspectives* 17, no.2 (March/April 1985): 90–96.

Luger, Harriett. *Lauren.* New York: Viking, 1979.

Mecklenburg, Marjory E., and Patricia G. Thompson. "The Adolescent Family Life Program as a Prevention Measure," *Public Health Reports* 98, no.1 (January/February 1983): 21–29.

Moore, Kristin A., and Martha R. Burt. *Private Crisis, Public Cost: Policy Perspectives on Teenage Childbearing.* Washington, DC: Urban Institute Press, 1982.

Oettinger, Katherine B., with Elizabeth C. Mooney. *"Not My Daughter": Facing Up to Adolescent Pregnancy.* Englewood Cliffs, NJ: Prentice-Hall, 1979.

Pittman, Karen, and Gina Adams. *An Advocate's Guide to Numbers.* Washington, DC: Children's Defense Fund, 1988.

Richards, Arlene Kramer, and Irene Willis. *What To Do If You or Someone You Know Is under 18 and Pregnant.* New York: Lothrop, Lee & Shepard, 1983.

U.S. House of Representatives. *Teen Pregnancy: What Is Being Done?: A State-by-State Look. 1985. A Report of the Select Committee on Children, Youth, and Families.* Washington, DC: U.S. Government Printing Office, 1986.

Wattleton, Faye. "American Teens: Sexually Active, Sexually Illiterate," *Journal of School Health* 57, no.9 (November 1987): 379–380.

Witt, Reni L., and Jeannine Masterson Michael. *Mom, I'm Pregnant: A Personal Guide for Teenagers.* New York: Stein and Day, 1982.

Resources
for Finding Out about Teenage Pregnancy

Teenage Pregnancy in Fiction

Included in this section are works of young-adult fiction that discuss teen pregnancy in some manner. The novels about teen pregnancy in this sampling were selected to provide a historical perspective as well as to represent the various options and considerations surrounding teen pregnancy.

Betancourt, Jeanne. **Sweet Sixteen and Never . . .** New York: Bantam, 1987. 136p.

Julie visits Planned Parenthood with her friend Gale, who is pregnant. Julie's mother discovers Julie's pills and confronts her. Julie angrily retorts that she knows her mother had a child when she was 16 and gave him up for adoption, after living in a dreary home for unwed mothers for six months.

Julie keeps Gale's pregnancy and subsequent abortion a secret and supports her friend through the abortion and the doubts she feels afterward. (Gale was initially very happy and relieved.) She even stands up to an antiabortion demonstrator they meet outside the clinic who tricks Gale into looking at her photographs of aborted fetuses, trying to dissuade her from her decision to abort.

Blume, Judy. **Forever.** Scarsdale, NY: Bradbury (Pocket Books), 1975. 220p.

In a subplot to this classic book about teenage sexuality, Katherine's friend Erica has a cousin, Sybil, who is pregnant and decides not to have an abortion because she wants the experience of giving birth. She gives the baby up for adoption, but is very sad.

Calvert, Patricia. **Stranger, You and I.** New York: Scribner's, 1987. 152p.

When 14-year-old Zee Crofton becomes pregnant by an acquaintance, her best friend, Hughie McBride, helps her to deal with her pregnancy. Zee resolves her pregnancy by living in a home for unwed mothers and then giving her child up for adoption. Written primarily from Hughie's point of view, this novel gives a male's perspective on the situation.

Cone, Molly. **Paul David Silverman Is a Father.** New York: Dutton Skinny Book, 1983. Black and white photographs by Harold Roth. 55p.

Teenagers Cathy and David get married when they learn they are expecting a baby. After they undergo unforeseen trials and adjustments, their baby is born, and they discover they are now a family.

Crutcher, Chris. **Chinese Handcuffs.** New York: Morrow, 1989. 202p.

Dillon Hemingway's brother Preston committed suicide. Preston's girlfriend, Stacy, leaves town without telling anyone she is carrying his child. When Stacy returns, her parents suddenly decide to adopt a baby. Dillon figures out who this baby really is, and Stacy makes a public announcement about the child's real parents.

Dizenzo, Patricia. **Phoebe.** New York: McGraw-Hill (Bantam), 1970. 120p.

At the age of 16, Phoebe realizes she is pregnant. Unable to tell her mother and father, Phoebe confides in her friends, who cannot help her. Desperate, she tells her boyfriend about her dilemma. The reader is left not knowing what happens to the unborn child.

Elfman, Blossom. **The Girls of Huntington House.** New York: Houghton Mifflin, 1972. 170p.

This book is based on the author's experiences as an English teacher in a home for unwed mothers, where she learns to understand the girls and their individual situations.

Elfman, Blossom. **A House for Jonnie O.** Boston: Houghton Mifflin, 1976. 175p.

Expectant teens Mary Anne, Ada, and Jonnie attempt to emancipate themselves by renting a broken-down house and moving in together. Ada, however, reunites with the father of her child and plans to leave. Realizing that they can no longer afford the rent if Ada leaves, the three young women decide to separate. Aware that hard times are ahead, Jonnie is comforted by the idea that all the choices she has made up to this point were her own. She contemplates the responsibilities of motherhood.

Eyerly, Jeannette. **Bonnie Jo, Go Home.** New York: Lippincott, 1972. 141p.

Written before abortions were federally legalized, this book tells the story of 16-year-old Bonnie Jo, who spends 11 days alone in New York City while she finds a doctor and arranges to get an abortion.

Eyerly, Jeannette. **A Girl Like Me.** New York: Lippincott (Berkley), 1966. 180p.

Robin, who has been adopted, stands by her friend Cass, who has decided to give her baby up for adoption. Robin also learns her true identity by searching for her birth mother.

Eyerly, Jeannette. **Someone To Love Me.** New York: Lippincott, 1987. 168p.

Flattered by the attentions of handsome, popular Lance Carter, Patrice, a 15-year-old latchkey child, "proves" her love by having sex with him when her mother is not home. When she gets pregnant, Lance drops her. Deciding to keep the baby, Patrice attends an alternative high school with a pregnant-teen program. With support from her mother, Patrice begins her life as a single parent. Her best friend, Lauren, remains helpful and loyal.

Hansen, Caryl. **I Think I'm Having a Baby.** New York: Avon, 1982. 109p.

Fifteen-year-old Laurie has secretly loved Peter Matthews for a long time. She takes advantage of being alone with Peter to show him how much she loves him, but then must consider the choices and problems she faces when she fears she is pregnant. Luckily, her fears are unrealized, but she discovers that promises made in the evening can be forgotten by the next day.

Head, Ann. **Mr. and Mrs. Bo Jo Jones.** New York: Putnam's, 1967. 189p.

July and Bo Jo marry as teens because July is pregnant. They face many hard and trying times and the loss of friends. When their baby dies, they decide to remain married and finish school.

Hinton, Nigel. **Getting Free.** Nashville, New York: Thomas Nelson, 1978. 190p.

Feeling pressure from their families, two English teenagers run away together when they discover they are expectant parents. Joann's father denounces them, so they flee to Scotland. Joann becomes ill and loses the baby. Peter decides that the relationship is over and suggests that they return home. Joann disagrees, so they continue as fugitives from the law.

Lee, Joanna. **I Want To Keep My Baby.** New York: New American Library, 1977. 166p.

Sue Ann is 15 and pregnant. Her boyfriend walks out on her, leaving her to raise the baby alone. Although she tries very hard to be a good mother, she is unable to make it on her own and relinquishes her baby for adoption because it was the best thing for her to do.

Lee, Mildred. **Sycamore Year.** New York: New American Library, 1974. 150p.

Wren's best friend, Anna, 15 and pregnant, turns to Wren for help. When Wren's plans to take Anna to her grandmother's farm fall through, Wren urges Anna to tell her mother about the pregnancy. Anna's mother is understanding and sends her to a home for unwed mothers. Anna finally decides on adoption and her mother supports her decision.

Lowry, Lois. **Rabble Starkey.** Boston: Houghton Mifflin, 1987. 192p.

Rabble's mother, Sweet-Hosanna, was a 14-year-old pregnant teenager whose husband left her when Rabble was one month old. When Sweet-Ho takes a job as a housekeeper for Mr. Bigelow, Rabble and her mother experience the security of a traditional family. But Sweet-Ho, having gained some confidence and education, wants to continue as a single parent.

Luger, Harriett. **Lauren.** New York: Viking (Dell), 1979. 176p.

Seventeen-year-old Lauren changes quickly from a carefree teen to an adult with burdens too great to bear. Disappointed with friends and family, she must decide among abortion, single parenthood, marriage, or adoption. Frustrated by the pressure to have an abortion, Lauren decides to continue the pregnancy. But she realizes the road is going to be rough and decides she must consider the best alternative for the baby. At the end of the book, Lauren remembers a childless couple she met and considers putting her baby up for adoption.

Madison, Winifred. **Growing Up in a Hurry.** New York: Little, Brown (Pocket Books), 1973. 200p.

Karen, 17, seems to have many emotional hangups, but when she meets Steve she feels great. She assures Steve she is safe from pregnancy, but actually puts off going to the clinic to get birth-control pills. When she tells Steve she is pregnant, he tells her to get an abortion. She decides that an abortion is the best decision for her. Her parents are upset but stand by her decision.

Miklowitz, Gloria D. **Unwed Mother.** New York: Tempo Books, 1977. 183p.

Kathy, 15, is trying to raise her baby at home but feels pressure from other family members. She meets two other teen mothers and they decide to find a place to rent together. Kathy realizes it is extremely hard to be a single parent and must face a final decision. After discussing adoption with her social worker, Kathy decides this would be best for her baby.

Neufeld, John. **For All the Wrong Reasons.** New York: New American Library, 1973. 220p.

Tish admires Peter and seduces him. They enjoy each other and continue their romance. When Tish discovers she is pregnant, she tells Peter she will get an abortion. Peter refuses to let her, saying he will marry her. After marriage and the birth of their baby, Peter feels detached from his friends and goes through a breakdown. Tish receives family support to raise the baby until Peter recovers.

Neufeld, John. **Sharelle.** New York: New American Library, 1983. 295p.

When 14-year-old Sharelle becomes pregnant by her future brother-in-law, her life is changed by her love and concern for her baby. While attending a school for teen parents, she decides adoption is the best answer for her.

Peck, Richard. **Don't Look and It Won't Hurt.** New York: Holt, Rinehart and Winston (Avon), 1979. 158p.

Ellen, 17 and unwed, has to leave home to have her baby. Her sister Carol comes and helps her make the decision to give the baby up for adoption. Although she never sees the baby, Ellen is satisfied just to know her child was healthy.

Prince, Alison. **The Turkey's Nest.** New York: Morrow, 1980. 223p.

Pregnant and unmarried, 17-year-old Kate leaves London to live with a distant relative. While living on the farm in Suffolk, Kate learns to enjoy country living. She marries a country boy and raises her baby on the farm.

Ruby, Lois. **What Do You Do in Quicksand?** New York: Viking, 1979. 199p.

Matt Russell, 16, can't give his baby daughter up for adoption after his girlfriend abandons her. He takes on the responsibility of raising his baby with the help of his parents and a neighbor friend, 15-year-old Leah.

Sherburne, Zoa. **Too Bad about the Haines Girl.** New York: Morrow, 1967. 184p.

Although out of print, this classic story about teenage pregnancy is acclaimed for its honest and straightforward approach.

Shreve, Susan. **Loveletters.** New York: Knopf, 1978. 217p.

Headstrong Kate finds life in a home for unwed mothers a stifling experience. She becomes ill with blood poisoning and has to have a cesarean section to ensure the baby's safety. The baby is fine, but Kate does not see the baby because she has decided to give him/her up for adoption. When she returns home, she must face the undesired attentions of a former playmate, now a mentally ill young man.

Stephensen, A. M. **Unbirthday.** New York: Flare, 1982. 112p.

After carefully researching the possibility of abortion, pregnant high school senior Louisa decides this is the best choice for her. A volunteer at the local women's center provides factual information and emotional support. Her boyfriend, Charlie, who is also a high school senior, remains loving, understanding, and supportive.

Trivelpiece, Laurel. **In Love and in Trouble.** New York: Pocket Books, 1981. 169p.

Sixteen-year-old Alma has admired Howard for a long time. When she gets the opportunity to be with him, she knows she must make the most of it. When she becomes pregnant she fears telling anyone. Howard wants her to have an abortion and sends her money to pay for it. She cannot go through with the abortion, but after she discovers how hard it is to raise the baby alone, she opts for adoption.

Truss, Jan. **Bird at the Window.** New York: Harper & Row, 1980. 215p.

When Angela Moynahan, the brain, discovers she is pregnant, she asserts her independence and goes to visit her grandmother in England. Angela decides to keep the baby, but it is stillborn. She returns home and, bolstered by the support of her former English teacher, Mr. Olson, focuses on her writing.

Zindel, Bonnie. **Hollywood Dream Machine.** New York: Viking (Bantam), 1984. 179p.

Seventeen-year-old Gabrielle Fuller spends the summer with her best friend, Buffy, whose family has moved from New York to California. Buffy's parents are very liberal and allow Zack to share Buffy's room on weekends. Buffy forgot to take her birth-control pills for four days and is now pregnant. She decides to have an abortion, and Gabrielle supports her as she carries out her decision. Buffy's story is only a minor part of this novel.

Zindel, Paul. **My Darling, My Hamburger.** New York: Harper & Row (Bantam), 1969. 122p.

Maggie and Liz seek acceptance from boys and other friends. They are faced with decisions about sex and resultant problems. When Liz's boyfriend, Sean, discovers that Liz is pregnant, he becomes furious and refuses to speak to her. Liz goes to the clinic and has an abortion. Only when she becomes ill do her parents learn about her pregnancy.

Nonfiction Materials on Teenage Pregnancy

The following nonfiction titles are mostly books, but some articles, pamphlets, and government documents are included. Because the number of publications on teenage pregnancy is large, this list is highly selective and primarily includes titles that are likely to be easily accessible in most major libraries and that will be readable and useful for young adults. Notations indicating the type of reader the publication is directed toward are added when appropriate.

BOOKS AND PAMPHLETS

Alan Guttmacher Institute. **Teenage Pregnancy: The Problem That Hasn't Gone Away.** New York: Alan Guttmacher Institute, 1981. 77p.

This publication provides a comprehensive overview of statistics and trends for teenage pregnancy in the 1970s. Information is provided through charts, graphs, and written commentaries. Black and white photographs are included.

Barr, Linda, and Catherine Monseratt. **Teenage Pregnancy: A New Beginning.** Edited by Caroline Gaston. Albuquerque: New Futures, 1978. 99p.

Written as the text for a family-life education course by teachers at a school for pregnant teens, this book covers the basics of human reproduction, sexual feelings, fetal development, sexually transmitted diseases, health care during pregnancy, choices, labor and delivery, newborn baby care, parenting, and family planning. Quotations, photographs, and case histories of students at New Futures School, plus drawings, a brief section devoted to teen fathers, and a glossary, make this book appealing, informative, and easy to read. A Spanish-English version is also available. Addressed specifically to pregnant teens, the book's tone is supportive, but matter-of-fact.

Bell, Ruth, et al. **Changing Bodies, Changing Lives: A Book for Teens on Sex and Relationships.** New York: Random House, 1987. 254p.

This comprehensive book on all aspects of teen sexuality and general health was written specifically for teenagers. Teens share their views on their sexual experiences. The authors write in a straightforward manner and provide a range of perspectives on each topic. Illustrations are particularly helpful in the sections on anatomy and contraception. This is one of the best resources available for teens.

Bode, Janet. **Kids Having Kids.** New York: Franklin Watts, 1980. 107p.

Geared to young adults, this book provides a historical perspective on pregnancy and sexual attitudes as well as information on contraceptives and options available to the pregnant teen. A bibliography is included.

Bowe-Gutman, Sonia. **Teen Pregnancy.** Minneapolis: Lerner, 1987. 71p.

Addressed to teenage readers, this book discusses values involving sexuality, the economics of child raising, health risks for teenage mothers and their babies, myths and facts of contraception, and parenting readiness. The author includes five case studies of pregnant teens, advice for teens who think they may be pregnant, and a list of organizations that provide information and counseling about pregnancy, birth control, family planning, and adoption.

Eagan, Andrea Boroff. **Why Am I So Miserable If These Are the Best Years of My Life?: Everything Your Mother Never Told You about Becoming a Woman.** New York: Avon, 1988. 211p.

Teenage pregnancy is one of the topics Eagan includes in this frank, honest, readable guide for young women. Her information is factual, but she does add her own opinions at times; for instance, she states that she considers abortion the best option for pregnant teens. Her background in the women's movement and the women's health movement are clearly evident.

Ewy, Donna, and Rodger Ewy. **Teen Pregnancy: The Challenges We Faced, the Choices We Made.** Boulder: Pruett, 1984, 188p.

Students in the Boulder Valley School teen-parenting class share their experiences of pregnancy, childbirth, and parenting. Interspersed with the girls' own stories is information about the first months of pregnancy, prenatal exams, prenatal care, childbirth, continuing school, job training, parenting choices, economic assistance, parenting practices, and contraception. Black and white photographs and drawings enhance the text.

Gates, Joanne, with help from Elizabeth McGee and Ruth Bell. "So You Think You Might Be Pregnant." In **Changing Bodies, Changing Lives: A Book for Teens on Sex and Relationships.** Ruth Bell, et al. New York: Random House, 1987. 194–222.

The authors direct this section to unmarried teenage girls and provide details about the signs of pregnancy, pregnancy tests, the role of the father, talking with parents, abortion, keeping the baby, foster care, and adoption. Quotations from interviews with pregnant teens are included.

Hayes, Cheryl D., ed. **Risking the Future: Adolescent Sexuality, Pregnancy, and Childbearing.** Vol. 1. Washington, DC: National Academy Press, 1987. 323p.

A summary of research done by the Committee on Child Development Research and Public Policy, this book contains some of the most up-to-date information on teen pregnancy. It was published by the National Research Council and is aimed primarily at researchers and policymakers. This scholarly book could be helpful to teachers.

McCoy, Kathy, and Charles Wibbelsman. **The New Teenage Body Book.** Los Angeles: Body Press, 1987. 278p.

Concerned with the overall health of teenagers, this handbook contains a chapter on teenage pregnancy and parenthood. Names and addresses of nationwide agencies that can help teenagers with health and sexual concerns are provided in the appendix. Illustrations and an index are also included. Readable and comprehensive, this handbook is an excellent resource for teenagers.

McGuire, Paula. **It Won't Happen to Me: Teenagers Talk about Pregnancy.** New York: Delacorte Press, 1983. 226p.

After a brief introduction to the problem of teen pregnancy, the author gives several in-depth case studies of pregnant girls. She also includes interviews with pregnant teens' physicians and social workers. The book covers diverse viewpoints on options for pregnant teens. It includes resource lists with important telephone numbers and addresses.

Miner, Jane Claypool. **Young Parents.** Black and white photography by Maureen McNicholas. New York: Julian Messner, 1985. 159p.

Written for the 3,000 teenagers who become pregnant every day, this book offers information to help young women make intelligent choices and take the responsibility for making them. Intertwined with the facts and statistics on teen pregnancy are the actual stories of pregnant teens, telling how they felt and what they did about their situations. The feelings of fathers and grandparents are also taken into consideration. A brief bibliography is included.

Moore, Kristin A., and Martha R. Burt. **Private Crisis, Public Cost: Policy Perspectives on Teenage Childbearing.** Washington, DC: Urban Institute Press, 1982. 166p.

This book brings together research done by the Urban Institute in an effort to change public policy. Written at a college level, this book would be most helpful to teachers or students needing extremely specific statistics. It includes an extensive bibliography.

Oettinger, Katherine B., with Elizabeth C. Mooney. **"Not *My* Daughter": Facing Up to Adolescent Pregnancy.** Englewood Cliffs, NJ: Prentice-Hall, 1979. 180p.

Written for the parents of pregnant teens, this book frankly discusses the facts and decisions surrounding teen pregnancy. The author is a psychiatric social worker internationally renowned for her work in social service. The book includes a resource guide to books, pamphlets, articles, films, and organizations that may be of further help to parents and professionals.

Richards, Arlene K., and Irene Willis. **What To Do If You or Someone You Know Is under 18 and Pregnant.** New York: Lothrop, Lee & Shepard, 1983. 250p.

Geared toward teenagers trying to make decisions about unplanned pregnancies, this book discusses the facts of sex, birth control, childbirth, abortion, adoption, and a little about raising a baby and the responsibilities of marriage.

The final chapter provides an annotated list of places and publications that can provide help for pregnant teens.

Vinovskis, Maris A. **An Epidemic of Teen Pregnancy? Some Historical and Policy Considerations.** New York: Oxford University Press, 1988. 253p.

Best used by a teacher or a very advanced student, this book examines whether there really is an "epidemic of teen pregnancy." The author discusses teen sexuality and pregnancy in a historical context and questions whether sex education is actually decreasing teen pregnancy. An extensive reference section is included.

Weston, Carol. **Girltalk about Guys.** New York: Harper & Row, 1988. 220p.

Structuring her information around real letters from teens, Weston devotes two-thirds of this book to topics relating to relationships. In the last section, she briefly discusses unwanted pregnancy and the options for teens. The information given is solid, and the advice shows a genuine caring for teens. The author's chatty style makes the information easy to read and her advice easy to accept.

Wharton, Mandy. **Understanding Social Issues: Abortion.** New York: Gloucester Press, 1989. 62p.

Written especially for young adults, this book presents both sides of the abortion issue. Personal dilemmas are presented along with historical, global, and social perspectives. Case studies, photographs, and illustrations enhance the text, and a glossary and index are provided. Examples and statistics from many countries make this a particularly worthwhile addition to the literature on abortion.

Witt, Reni L., and Jeannine Masterson Michael. **Mom, I'm Pregnant: A Personal Guide for Teenagers.** New York: Stein and Day, 1982. 230p.

Written specifically for pregnant teens, this book provides moral support as well as factual information. The text explores several options: abortion, adoption, foster care, marriage, and living with the father. One of the authors is a social worker who has worked directly with pregnant teens. The book includes an extensive bibliography and state-by-state hotline numbers.

ARTICLES

Berman, Claire. **"Teenage Pregnancy: A Grandmother Too Soon!"** *McCall's* (May 1987): 84–86.

Mothers of teen mothers explain the anger, disappointment, and resentment they experienced over their daughters' pregnancies. They discuss the circumstances that surround incorporating a baby into the existing family structure, the sacrifices they make as grandmothers, and the love and pride they feel, despite their wishes that they had never been put in such situations.

Van Gelder, Lindsy, and Pam Brandt. **"Teenage Pregnancy: The Crisis in America."** *McCall's* (May 1987): 83.

In this brief introduction to a special report published in the same issue, the authors provide an overview of the statistics associated with teenage pregnancy.

Nonprint Materials on Teenage Pregnancy

The selections included in this list come from a variety of sources, including *Lander's Film Review*, Planned Parenthood video selections, and *School Library Booklist*. The selections here express a wide variety of viewpoints on the subject of teen pregnancy.

And Baby Makes Two: A Look at Teenage Single Parents
Type: VHS or Beta videocassette
Length: 25 min.
Cost: Rental $50; purchase $260

Distributor: Center Communications
12801 Schabarum Avenue
P.O. Box 7878
Irwindale, CA 91706
Date: 1986

Teen parents discuss the way their lives have been affected by the addition of a child. The reasons why one million teenage girls get pregnant every year are examined. This film recommends explicit sex and birth-control education, an emphasis on male responsibilities, and legislation that promotes responsible sexual and family habits.

Another Half
Type: 16mm film, VHS videocassette
Length: 27 min.
Cost: Rental $50; purchase $495 (film), $395 (video)
Distributor: Bill Wadsworth Productions
1913 W. 37th
Austin, TX 78731
Date: 1985

This film presents the thoughts of a high school boy about recent events involving a friend and a pregnant girl.

Children of Children
Type: 16mm film, VHS videocassette
Length: 30 min.
Cost: Purchase $550 (film), $450 (video)
Distributor: Coronet/MTI Film and Video
108 Wilmot Road
Deerfield, IL 60015
Date: 1988

Collin Siedor hosts this film that discusses the social and economic effects of teenage pregnancy.

Four Pregnant Teenagers: Four Different Decisions
Type: 35mm film, VHS videocassette
Length: 51 min.
Cost: Rental $95; purchase $209 (film), $249 (video)

Distributor: Sunburst Communications
Room RB36
101 Castleton Street
Pleasantville, NY 10570-3498
Date: 1988

These true-life stories dramatize the financial and emotional problems that unwed pregnant teens face and point out the options available to the pregnant teenager.

"I Never Thought It Would Be Like This": Teenagers Speak Out about Being Pregnant/Being Parents
Type: VHS videocassette
Length: 50 min.
Cost: Purchase $209
Distributor: Guidance Associates, Inc.
Communications Park, Box 3000
Mt. Kisco, NY 10549
Date: 1987

Through personal interviews with teenage girls, this video examines the physical, emotional, and social consequences an accidental pregnancy has on the mother, father, and child.

I Think I'm Having a Baby
Type: 16mm film, VHS videocassette
Length: 29 min.
Cost: Rental $75; purchase $500 (film), $250 (video)
Distributor: Coronet/MTI Film and Video
108 Wilmot Road
Deerfield, IL 60015
Date: 1982

In the context of an adult-living class for high school students, statistics about pregnancy are presented. One student in the class fears she is pregnant, but later discovers she is not.

Is That What You Want for Yourself?
Type: 16mm film, VHS videocassette
Length: 13 min.

Cost:	Rental $50; purchase $250 (film), $200 (video)
Distributor:	Coronet/MTI Film and Video
108 Wilmot Road
Deerfield, IL 60015
Date:	1980

This film focuses on a 15-year-old who believes she is pregnant and is suddenly faced with numerous decisions concerning her future. It invites discussion by ending with her choice undecided.

It Only Takes Once

Type:	VHS Videocassette
Length:	18 min.
Cost:	Purchase $189.95
Distributor:	Intermedia
1300 Dexter Avenue North
Seattle, WA 98109
Date:	1986

With Danitra Vance, formerly of "Saturday Night Live," as host, several teens discuss their feelings and pressures regarding sex, contraceptives, and babies. Teen couples with babies describe their lives as teen parents. This video stresses that saying no is an option.

Life with Baby

Type:	16mm film, VHS videocassette
Length:	27 min.
Cost:	Rental $55; purchase $500 (film), $295 (video)
Distributor:	Filmakers Library
124 E. 40th Street
New York, NY 10016
Date:	1985

The focus is on the frustrations and problems that come from being a teenage parent.

A Matter of Love

Type:	VHS videocassette
Length:	43 min.
Cost:	Rental $35; purchase $295

Distributor: Perennial Education, Inc.
930 Pitner Avenue
Evanston, IL 60202
Date: 1986

This video illustrates the emotional turmoil experienced by a young, unwed pregnant couple and a married couple who are unable to conceive. An interesting parallel is drawn as the teenage couple decides putting the baby up for adoption will ensure them all a brighter future and the married couple decides adopting a baby will bring them a brighter future.

Me, a Teen Father?
Type: 16mm film, VHS videocassette
Length: 13 min.
Cost: Rental $50; purchase $325 (film), $235 (video)
Distributor: Coronet/MTI Film and Video
Dist. of LCA
108 Wilmot Road
Deerfield, IL 60015
Date: 1980

A look at the problems and emotions a teenage father must face.

Mother, May I?
Type: 16mm film, VHS videocassette
Length: 28 min.
Cost: Rental $60; purchase $480 (film), $335 (video)
Distributor: Churchill Films
12210 Nebraska Avenue
Los Angeles, CA 90025
Date: 1982

A pregnancy scare is the basis for this story about a family groping for communication in the face of their 16-year-old daughter's budding sexuality.

People Who Have Struggled with Abortion
Type: 16mm film, VHS videocassette
Length: 29 min.
Cost: Rental $65 (film), $50 (video); purchase $450 (film), $300 (video)

Distributor: Martha Stuart Communications
147 W. 22nd Street
New York, NY 10011
Date: 1981

In an honest, open discussion, people from all walks of life who have struggled with abortion discuss the philosophic, religious, and legal issues involved.

Pregnant Teens: Taking Care
Type: 16mm film, VHS videocassette
Length: 22 min.
Cost: Rental $45; purchase $450
Distributor: Perennial Education, Inc.
930 Pitner Avenue
Evanston, IL 60202
Date: 1983

Two pregnant teens, one black and one white, are going through a prenatal class. They share similar feelings about their pregnancies. The emphasis is on providing complete prenatal care information.

Real People: Meet a Teenage Mother
Type: 35mm film, VHS videocassette
Length: 18 min.
Cost: Rental $55; purchase $109 (film), $145 (video)
Distributor: Sunburst Communications
Room RB36
101 Castleton Street
Pleasantville, NY 10570-3498
Date: 1988

Lauri, 17, discusses the problems faced by a single young mother.

Schoolboy Father
Type: 16mm film, VHS videocassette
Length: 30 min.
Cost: Rental $75; purchase $500 (film), $250 (video)
Distributor: Coronet/MTI Film and Video
108 Wilmot Road
Deerfield, IL 60015
Date: 1981

Based on a novel by Jeannette Eyerly, *He's My Baby Now*, this is the story of a father who, after discovering he has fathered a child, wants to keep it against the mother's wishes. After a week's trial period of living with the child, he agrees to give it up for adoption.

Shelley & Pete (. . . & Carol)
Type: VHS or Beta videocassette
Length: 23 min.
Cost: Purchase $110
Distributor: National Audio Visual Center
8700 Edgeworth Drive
Capitol Heights, MA 20743
Date: 1981

Shelley becomes pregnant and marries Pete, and this high school couple faces economic and emotional hardships.

So Many Voices: A Look at Abortion in America
Type: 16mm film, VHS videocassette
Length: 30 min.
Cost: Rental $50; purchase $475 (film), $275 (video)
Distributor: Phoenix Films & Video
468 Park Avenue South
New York, NY 10016
Date: 1982

Actors Ed Asner and Tammy Grimes host this film, which uses testimonials and current film clips to explore both sides of the abortion issue.

Teen Mother—A Story of Coping
Type: VHS videocassette
Length: 24 min.
Cost: Rental $60; purchase $440 (film), $310 (video)
Distributor: Mobius Production Ltd.
Churchill Films
12210 Nebraska Avenue
Los Angeles, CA 90025
Date: 1985

This is a documentary about the everyday life of a young single mother.

Teenage Father
Type: VHS videocassette
Length: 38 min.
Cost: Rental $75; purchase $205
Distributor: Sunburst Communication
Room RB36
101 Castleton Street
Pleasantville, NY 10570-3498
Date: 1989

A focus on three young men shows the anxiety, confusion, and guilt that teenage fathers often suffer.

Teenage Mother: Beyond the Baby Shower
Type: VHS videocassette
Length: 27 min.
Cost: Rental $35; purchase $295
Distributor: Perennial Education, Inc.
930 Pitner Avenue
Evanston, IL 60602
Date: 1988

By emphasizing the decision-making process, this program encourages teens to make thoughtful, informed decisions regarding their sexuality. Three middle-class rural women discuss the realities of teen parenthood and their desire to do it all over again. They stress that saying no is a completely acceptable option.

Teenage Parents, Their Lives Have Changed
Type: 16mm film, VHS videocassette
Length: 23 min.
Cost: Rental $60; purchase $495 (film), $395 (video)
Distributor: Alfred Higgins Productions
6350 Laurel Canyon Boulevard
North Hollywood, CA 91601
Date: 1987

Several teens show how their lives changed after they became parents, emphasizing that parenthood can be exhausting and demanding.

Teenage Pregnancy: No Easy Answers
Type: 16mm film, VHS or Beta videocassette
Length: 22 min.
Cost: Rental $50; purchase $495 (film), $345 (video)
Distributor: Barr Films
12801 Schabarum Avenue
P.O. Box 7878
Irwindale, CA 91706
Date: 1980

A 15-year-old girl discovers she is pregnant and thinks through many options. The film ends before she makes her decision and is designed to stimulate class discussion on decision making.

The Teenage Pregnancy Experience
Type: 16mm film, VHS videocassette
Length: 26 min.
Cost: Rental $48; purchase $370 (film), $315 (video)
Distributor: Parenting Pictures
121 NW Crystal Street
Crystal River, FL 32629
Date: 1981

Pregnant teenagers and school-age parents discuss the choices they made regarding unplanned pregnancies and why they did not use birth control in the first place.

Teens Having Babies
Type: 16mm film, VHS videocassette
Length: 20 min.
Cost: Rental $40; purchase $395 (film), $295 (video)
Distributor: Polymorph Films, Inc.
118 South Street
Boston, MA 02111
Date: 1983

This practical film shows the steps a teen mother goes through after becoming pregnant. It explains visits to hospitals, prenatal care, and delivery techniques.

When Teens Get Pregnant

Type: 16mm film, VHS videocassette
Length: 19 min.
Cost: Rental $40; purchase $395 (film), $295 (video)
Distributor: Polymorph Films
118 South Street
Boston, MA 02111
Date: 1982

Interviews with several pregnant teens show the physical and emotional pain involved with teenage pregnancy.

Young Fathers: Teenage Love

Type: VHS videocassette
Length: 12 min.
Cost: Rental $40; purchase $245
Distributor: New Dimension Films
85895 Lorane Highway
Eugene, OR 97405
Date: 1985

Three dramatic scenes about teenage fatherhood are presented to promote classroom discussion.

Organizations Concerned with Teenage Pregnancy

There are many agencies to help deal with teen pregnancy. Some are organized at a national level, while others are locally based. The first place to check is in your local Yellow Pages. You might look under Birth Control Information, Churches, Clergy, Clinics, Counseling, Crisis Intervention Services, Family Planning, Marriage Counselors, Mental Health Services, Psychiatrists, Psychologists, and Social Service Organizations.

Telephone numbers with an 800 prefix indicate there is no long-distance charge for the call.

Child Welfare League of America
440 First Street, NW, Suite 310
Washington, DC 20001
(202) 638-2952

Executive Director: David S. Liederman

The Child Welfare League of America is an association of child-welfare agencies in the United States and Canada. Its main offices are in Washington, D.C. There is a special program for adolescent pregnancy, and the staff can connect you with agencies that offer pregnancy counseling and adoption services.

PUBLICATIONS: Books and pamphlets.

Federation of Feminist Women's Health Centers
6221 Wilshire Boulevard, Suite 419
Los Angeles, CA 90048
(213) 469-4844
Director: Carol Downer

This agency provides information and services such as well-woman clinics, family counseling, abortions, birth control, and safe sex. It offers telephone counseling and referrals. Although centers associated with the Federation of Feminist Women's Health Centers are located primarily in California, Georgia, and Washington, the Los Angeles office can refer you to similar services in your area. If you don't have the money, try calling collect.

PUBLICATIONS: Women's self-help information.

The Gladney Center
2300 Hemphill Street
Fort Worth, TX 76110
(800) GLA-DNEY
Director: Michael J. McMahon

The Gladney Center is a residential home for pregnant girls waiting to have a baby. Most give their babies up for adoption, but this is not a prerequisite. Programs available through the Gladney Center include residential, nonresidential, medical, educational, recreational, spiritual, counseling, and infant-placement services. Fees are based on the client's ability to pay. No one is turned away because of lack of financial resources.

PUBLICATIONS: *Ours* (quarterly newsletter), brochures.

March of Dimes, National Headquarters
600 Third Avenue
New York, NY 10017
(914) 428-7100
Deputy Director for Community Services: Ann McGovern

March of Dimes staff and volunteers are available to conduct seminars about teenage pregnancy. Contact your local chapter for more information.

PUBLICATIONS: Videotapes and handouts about teenage pregnancy.

Planned Parenthood Federation of America
810 Seventh Avenue
New York, NY 10019
(212) 541-7800
President: Faye Wattleton

Planned Parenthood Federation of America, Inc., is the nation's oldest and largest voluntary family-planning organization. It began with the first birth-control clinic in America, founded in 1916 by Margaret Sanger. Planned Parenthood is dedicated to the principle that every individual has the fundamental right to choose when or whether to have children. Services provided by local chapters include pregnancy diagnosis, abortion counseling and referrals, prenatal care, and infertility treatment. Consult your local phone book for the Planned Parenthood clinic nearest you.

PUBLICATIONS: Pamphlets on a variety of reproductive health-care topics.

Hotline

Adoption Hotline   (202) 328-8072
Calling this hotline will put you in contact with an operator who will provide information about local and out-of-state adoption agencies or pregnancy services.

CHAPTER 5

Sexually Transmitted Diseases

"I had it once."

We stopped walking and dropped hands. "You had VD?"

"I got it from this girl in Maine . . . the only time I ever got laid.

"You've only been laid once?"

"Well, twice . . . but with the same girl."

"That's all?"

"What do you mean, *that's all?* What'd you expect?"

"I don't know. . . . I thought you had lots of experience."

"Yeah, well . . . the clap turned me off for a while."

"I can imagine," I said. We started walking again, this time without holding hands. "Did you tell the girl in Maine?"

"I couldn't. . . . I didn't even know her last name. She was just somebody I met on the beach."
Judy Blume, Forever (Scarsdale, NY:
Bradbury, 1975), 90–91.

Michael, in Judy Blume's novel *Forever*, loves Katherine and is becoming sexually intimate with her. Telling her he once had VD, or the venereal disease called gonorrhea (the clap), is part of their growing sexual intimacy. It is also a responsible thing to do, even though he is now cured and he will never see his casual sex partner again.

> "AIDS?!" I shivered. "I . . . I don't understand. It can't be!"
>
> And he told me all about the visits to Dr. Hoff, the blood tests and results, and how he no doubt caught it through the transfusions. "So, you see, I don't exactly have AIDS, but I've been exposed to the virus and developed AIDS Related Complex. And I could get AIDS—there's a twenty to thirty percent chance."
>
> Without realizing it I'd moved away from Alex so my back was pressing against the door handle.
>
> "The worst of it is—I may have infected *you!*" he cried at last, in anguish. "It kills me to think that!"
>
> I'd heard so much so fast that it didn't really sink in until these last words. And now that it did, all I could do was stare at him and shudder.
>
> "How?" I whispered. "We used precaution."
>
> "Sure, so you wouldn't get pregnant. Not to prevent AIDS. Who would have thought you'd have been better off if we'd not switched to the pill."
>
> He took my hands in his and peered solemnly into my eyes. "You know I'd never do anything to hurt you!"
>
> Gloria D. Miklowitz, *Good-bye Tomorrow* (New York: Delacorte, 1987), 99–100.

Alex in Gloria Miklowitz's *Good-bye Tomorrow* has only recently learned he has ARC, AIDS-related complex, and now he must tell his girlfriend she may have contracted the virus from him. Alex is not gay. He and Shannon have had intercourse only with each other. But he was in an automobile accident and had two blood transfusions before the medical community knew to test for the AIDS virus in donated blood. So the blood that saved Alex's life also infected him with the AIDS virus.

"Does Jim know you have this thing?" I asked him.

"Say AIDS, Ricky," Pete said. "Mom and Dad are calling it a thing, a bug, everything but AIDS. . . . Yes, Jim knows. We were both sick all through Europe. I kept telling myself I had what he had, some kind of dysentery. But my lymph nodes were swollen, and I had these little red spots on my ankles. I had all these explanations to myself for what they were. But I couldn't ever get my strength back, and there were more spots. I began to really panic by the time I came out to Seaville last time. Mom wanted me to go see Doctor Rapp there. By then I had this big purple bruise under my arm. When I saw that, I began to face the fact I could have AIDS."

M. E. Kerr, Night Kites (New York:
Harper & Row, 1986), 98.

Pete in M. E. Kerr's *Night Kites* does indeed have AIDS. He is homosexual and has had multiple sex partners. By the time he tells his brother Eric (Ricky) about it, Pete has come to terms with his inevitable death. Pete's family had not known he was gay, but they adjust to this information and support Pete completely.

Members of the community, however, harbor misinformation about the disease. The family's housekeeper leaves after 20 years of service; Eric's girlfriend, Nicki, is forbidden to see him because it would be bad for her father's motel business; and Nicki herself thinks Eric could have given her the virus since his brother has AIDS. Even one of Pete's gay friends refuses to see him—although his other friends, particularly Jim, are quite supportive.

AIDS, its precursor ARC, and gonorrhea are among the sexually transmitted diseases (STDs) that have reached epidemic proportions in the United States during this century. Like the characters in these novels, many young people these days are affected in one way or another by STDs. Teens who have not contracted an STD themselves may have a friend or relative who has, or may at some time become sexually intimate with someone who may infect them with an STD.

- Sexually transmitted diseases (other than AIDS) constitute the most widespread epidemic in North America (Eagan, 144).
- "The age group at highest risk for STDs includes individuals between 10 and 19 years old" (National Institute of Allergy and Infectious Diseases, 1).
- "Approximately 2.5 million teenagers are affected with a sexually transmitted disease each year" (U.S. Department of Health and Human Services, 110).

Because STDs are so widespread, it is important to understand how to prevent their spread and to be aware of possible cures, should they be contracted.

What Is an STD?

Sexually transmitted disease (STD) is the term used for what used to be called a venereal disease. In its broad sense, a venereal disease is any disease passed through sexual contact. But the term venereal disease, or VD, acquired a limited meaning in common usage, so many people thought VD referred only to gonorrhea or syphilis. STD is the term we now use to identify any disease passed from one person to another through sexual contact. Sexual contact can mean kissing, making out, or having any form of intercourse—vaginal, oral, or anal. Some STDs can be transmitted through other means as well.

Signs of STDs

Although each STD has particular signs and symptoms, which will be described below, there are some general indicators that an STD may be present. Any unusual discharge from a girl's vagina could be a sign of an STD. A normal vaginal discharge is the blood shed during her menstrual period or the white or clear mucus that is part of the vagina's self-cleansing process. An abnormal discharge might be a yellowish pus, indicating infection. Sores, warts, or itching in her genital area, rashes on her hands or feet, burning urination, and lower abdominal pain may also be symptoms of STDs.

A clear or white discharge from a boy's penis could signal an STD, as could sores around the penis or anus, burning urination, itching in the genital area, rashes on the hands and feet, or a pain in the groin.

When an STD Is Suspected

Any suspicion of an STD should be followed up by a medical examination as soon as possible. Clinics are generally prepared to deal with people with STDs. Charges will vary according to the clinic and sometimes the patient's ability to pay. State boards of health or departments of health provide free STD tests and treatment. Private doctors can also test and treat for STDs. All medical facilities are legally required to keep visits confidential, but the law does require they report the number of incidents of STDs in an effort to curb the spread of these diseases.

During the medical exam, the health professional examines the patient for sores, rashes, swellings, and infections. Blood tests, culture tests, and Gram's stain tests will be administered to determine the existence of STDs.

Blood test. A blood test involves taking a sample of blood from the patient's arm and sending the sample to a laboratory where it is tested for various STD antibodies. The presence of these antibodies indicates the disease has infected the patient's body.

Culture test. A culture test involves using a cotton swab to remove a sample from the infected area of the body. A boy would have samples taken from his penis, anus, and throat. A girl would have them taken from her cervix, anus, and throat. Each sample is placed on a culture dish where it must grow for 16 to 24 hours or longer. Then it is analyzed for STDs.

Gram's stain test. The Gram's stain test involves taking a sample of discharge, putting it on a slide, and examining it under the microscope.

Test results tell the health professional if STDs are present and if treatment is necessary. Paying attention to unusual signs on one's body and having a medical exam can expedite this process. Ignoring STD symptoms is dangerous and can lead to sterility (the inability to have children) or even death.

Tests When No Symptoms Are Present

Unfortunately, not everyone infected with an STD manifests symptoms that signal the presence of the disease. Females in particular can have an STD like gonorrhea and not show signs for a long time. Unnoticed, the disease continues to spread throughout the girl's reproductive system and she may become permanently sterile. Anyone with whom an infected girl has intercourse is at high risk for contracting that disease.

Because she may have an STD and not know it, a sexually active girl needs to be tested for STDs once a year. These tests can be easily administered during the regular gynecological examination, which doctors recommend for all sexually active girls anyway. (See Chapter 3.) She may also choose to have only the tests done.

Girls having sex with several different people, or with a partner who has several other partners, would be well advised to have STD tests twice a year. Boys can, of course, also have STD testing during their annual physicals.

Responsibilities

Having sexual relations during an STD epidemic demands certain responsibilities.

PREVENTION

Obviously, abstaining from sexual intercourse is one certain way to avoid STDs. However, having intercourse with only one partner who does not have other partners is a fairly safe risk, providing neither person came into the relationship with an existing STD. Knowing the personal health record of one's sexual partner(s) is important and necessitates honest communication; it often precludes casual sex. Observing potential sex partners for STD symptoms and avoiding sexual contact with those who have genital sores or abnormal discharges can also help one avoid STDs.

Using a contraceptive that protects against STDs is also highly recommended. Foam and condoms is the combination that most medical experts recommend. The foam contains a spermicide that kills many STD germs, and the condom prevents semen that may be carrying STD germs from entering the girl's vagina and cervix. The condom also protects the boy's penis from STD germs the girl may be harboring. Together they function as backup systems not only for preventing the passing of STDs, but for preventing pregnancy as well.

COMMUNICATION

Honesty with one's sexual partners is imperative. This means that if a boy discovers he has an STD, he must tell all his sexual partners so they may be tested for the disease. This is the only way some women discover they are STD carriers.

Although it is universally advised that anyone having a known STD should abstain from sexual relations, STD-infected people who choose to remain sexually active must tell their sex partners the risk they are taking. In addition, anyone having multiple sex partners or having intercourse with someone who has other sex partners should seriously consider taking precautions against STDs, both for their own health and to prevent further spread of STDs.

TREATMENT

It is essential that anyone infected with an STD receive treatment as soon as possible. Couples with STDs should be treated simultaneously so they do not continue to pass the STD back and forth even though one may be treated and cured.

Types of STDs

VIRUSES

A virus is an infinitesimally small microorganism that lives independently. A virus invades a human body cell, making the cell produce more viruses. The cell is ultimately destroyed, and the virus then moves on to another cell. This cell-destroying process repeats itself, putting the whole organism at risk. Fortunately, the body's immune system can effectively fight off most viruses. Unfortunately, some of the viruses it cannot fight off are STD viruses.

Genital herpes. Genital herpes results in painful sores that appear on or in the penis, vagina, and/or anus. They are caused by the highly infectious herpes simplex Type 2 virus. This virus is very similar to the herpes simplex Type 1 virus, which causes cold sores or fever blisters around the mouth. Once a herpes virus invades a human cell, it remains in that person's body for the rest of his or her life. The number of people harboring the Type 2 genital herpes virus has reached epidemic proportions in the United States.

- "In 1987, nearly 25 percent of the adult population in the U.S. was believed to be infected with the herpes simplex virus" (National Institute of Allergy and Infectious Diseases, 5).
- Seventy-five percent of people with herpes do not develop symptoms and are unaware they are infected but can still transmit the disease (ibid.).
- There are approximately 500,000 new cases of genital herpes every year (Nourse, 24).
- Genital herpes is by far the fastest-spreading STD in the United States (ibid.).
- "The high incidence of primary infections begins to appear at the age at which young people become sexually active—around twelve on up—and continues appearing into young adulthood (ibid., 30).

Everyone with genital herpes has had at least one episode with herpes sores and may have had recurring incidents as well. The symptoms of a first episode begin to show two to twenty days after the virus invades the body. The spot that was exposed to the virus is very sensitive and has a tingling, numb, itchy, and/or burning sensation. Within a few hours red marks appear at the site of the exposure. These red marks turn into painful, fluid-filled blisters. The infected person may also experience swollen lymph glands, general muscle aches, and an overall sick feeling.

In a day or so, the blisters develop into raw, moist, painful open sores. After about two weeks, these open sores scab over and begin to heal. The healing process takes ten to eleven days. When the sores are healed, the active virus is gone. This first episode of genital herpes usually lasts around four weeks. After the episode is over, the virus travels to the collection of nerve endings at the base of the skull where it remains dormant or inactive until the next eruption of sores. Recurrent episodes are usually less severe and shorter in duration.

Genital herpes is transmitted by skin-to-skin contact. A person showing any of the genital herpes symptoms—from itching to scabbing—is contagious, but the open-sore stage is the most highly infectious. When a person has direct contact with the infected area of another person's body, through touching, kissing, and other forms of sexual contact, he or she will in all likelihood acquire the herpes virus.

Furthermore, because Type 1 and Type 2 herpes viruses are almost identical, oral-genital contact with someone who has a cold sore (Type 1) can result in genital herpes infection (Type 2) (Gulas and Griffiths, 6). A person can also spread the herpes virus from one part of his or her own body to another after touching the infected area. In addition, a baby can acquire genital herpes if the herpes virus is present in the mother's birth canal.

The best way to prevent the spread of genital herpes is to avoid any sexual contact with anyone who has genital sores. Oral contact with anyone who has sores around his or her mouth should also be avoided. The next best way is for the boy to wear a condom during intercourse, although the virus is so small it can pass through the condom itself. Spermicidal foams, creams, and jellies are ineffective against the herpes virus. Although the virus cannot live for more than about two hours outside the host, it is wise to avoid using towels or other articles known to have been in contact with the body of anyone infected with herpes sores.

A culture test or a Pap smear, which are part of a gynecological exam (see Chapter 3), are usually used to identify the presence of the genital herpes virus. Although there is no cure for genital herpes, it is important that a doctor examine anyone who suspects he or she may have herpes. If the Type 2 herpes virus is discovered early in the first episode, it can be treated with Zovirax ointment or oral acyclovir to reduce the severity of the initial and recurring attacks. It is critical that a health professional monitor the pregnancy of anyone infected with the herpes virus.

AIDS. Acquired immune deficiency syndrome (AIDS) is the newest viral STD. Most teens have heard of it by now, but before 1981 it was a virtually unknown disease. AIDS has received extensive media coverage in an effort to educate the public about this rapidly spreading new disease that has claimed the lives of so many people.

- About 83,000 cases of AIDS had been reported in the United States by the end of 1988 (Centers for Disease Control quoted in Hein, 25).
- By the end of 1987, 56 percent of the 50,000 people with AIDS in the United States had died (U.S. Department of Health and Human Services, 10).
- The U.S. Public Health Service predicts that by the end of 1991, approximately 270,000 AIDS cases will have occurred in the United States (Langone, 67).
- According to U.S. Public Health Service estimates, 179,000 people will have died of AIDS by the end of 1991 (ibid.).

In 1988 there were 800 reported cases of AIDS for people between the ages of 13 and 21 (Hein, 6). Compared to the total number of AIDS cases, this figure may seem small and may seem to indicate that teens are not at risk for AIDS. It must be remembered, however, that AIDS often takes years to develop after a person has been exposed. Teens infected with the virus may not develop AIDS until they are in their 20s.

The AIDS infection begins when the AIDS virus (which is called the human immunodeficiency virus or HIV) invades the body and attacks the cells of its immune system. The immune system tries to protect the body against the HIV by producing antibodies to fight it off. However, these antibodies are ineffective in ridding the body of HIV and the HIV remains. The HIV slowly destroys the cells in the immune system, making that person defenseless against the infections and diseases an otherwise healthy person would normally fight off.

The invasion of HIV is the first step in the development of AIDS, but everybody who has been infected with HIV does not necessarily develop AIDS. There are often no symptoms at this stage, although the person may feel tired and have swollen glands. A blood test at this point would be termed HIV-positive, because it would show the presence of HIV antibodies. A person with such a blood test is referred to as HIV-infected.

ARC, or AIDS-related complex, is the intermediate step in the development of AIDS. Symptoms of ARC may include swollen glands, loss of more than ten pounds in less than two months, night sweats, fever, diarrhea, dry coughing, white spots or sores on the tongue or in the mouth or vagina, skin rashes, tiredness, and lack of resistance to infection. These symptoms indicate the immune system is seriously weakened.

Full-blown AIDS (often called just AIDS) is the final stage in this progression. Patients are diagnosed as having AIDS if they are HIV-positive and they develop one or more life-threatening opportunistic diseases. An opportunistic disease is caused by a virus that takes advantage of the fact that the immune system is functioning improperly. A person with a normally functioning immune system would not be affected by these diseases. The appearance of such an opportunistic disease indicates the immune system is severely deficient.

Two examples of opportunistic diseases are Kaposi's sarcoma and dementia. Kaposi's sarcoma is a rare form of cancer. Dementia is a form of mental deterioration that may lead to insanity. Opportunistic diseases are fatal.

Because the HIV or AIDS virus starts the process that leads to full-blown AIDS, it is important to understand how it is transmitted. Anyone who is HIV-positive can transmit the AIDS virus. An AIDS virus can be passed through body fluids like blood, semen, saliva, or tears. Semen, blood, and vaginal fluids are particularly effective transmission agents.

Sexual contact of any type—vaginal, oral, or anal—can transmit the AIDS virus. Anal intercourse can be particularly risky because the multitude of delicate blood vessels around the anus and in the rectum can be easily broken, providing an open wound where infected semen and blood can intermingle. Both homosexual and heterosexual sex partners are susceptible to the AIDS virus, but currently in the United States more gay or bisexual men have developed AIDS. However, the incidence of AIDS among heterosexual couples is rising.

Intravenous (IV) drug users can also transmit the AIDS virus when an infected user shares his or her contaminated needle with someone else. Transfusions with HIV-contaminated blood can also spread the virus, but this happens rarely now since all donors are screened and blood donations are carefully tested. The AIDS virus can also be passed to babies as a mother's infected blood flows into the placenta during pregnancy or in the birth canal during delivery. In addition, the virus can be transmitted through breast milk while the child nurses. Of all the types of blood transmissions, those from IV drug users are the most frequent.

Transmission of the AIDS virus can be prevented by not sharing an IV needle and avoiding any type of sexual contact with anyone who could possibly be infected with the AIDS virus. Abstinence is the only 100 percent guarantee of safety from sexual transmission. However, if one chooses not to abstain from sex, condoms can help, but they are only 90 percent effective, and that 10 percent risk is unwise when the stakes are so great. Adding a spermicidal foam to condom use can increase its effectiveness against the AIDS virus, but this is still not 100 percent safe. Engaging in sexual activities, like petting and mutual masturbation, that do not involve the exchange of body fluids is safer than having sexual intercourse (Hein, 40–41).

Testing for the AIDS virus begins with a blood test called an enzyme-linked immunosorbent assay (ELISA), which indicates the presence of HIV antibodies, showing the person is infected with the AIDS virus. A positive ELISA is followed up with a Western blot test for confirmation of the AIDS virus.

These tests can be administered through most doctors' offices and clinics. The blood samples will be sent to a laboratory for analysis. In some areas, the law requires that the names of all HIV-positive people be reported to health officials. AIDS testing can cost from $20 to $150, depending on the city and type of health facility used.

Once a person has been infected with HIV, there is no way to prevent the eventual onset of AIDS, and AIDS is fatal.

- Three out of ten HIV-infected people will develop AIDS sometime within five years (ibid., 10–11).
- Five out of seven HIV-infected people will develop AIDS sometime within seven years (ibid.).

When the HIV infection has weakened the immune system, it is wise to take good care of oneself and try to avoid infectious situations. All sexual contact must be eliminated, even with other people diagnosed as HIV-positive. Exposure to more contaminated body fluids can intensify the situation. It is imperative to notify all previous sex partners that they may have contracted the AIDS virus.

Hepatitis B. Hepatitis B is a viral disease that attacks the liver. Symptoms of hepatitis B are much like those of the flu and include nausea, muscle achiness, fatigue, fever, loss of appetite, headaches, and dizziness. In some cases the infected person's urine will become darker, stools will become lighter, eyes and skin will appear yellow, and the liver will feel tender. The symptoms appear between one and six months after contact with the hepatitis B virus.

The hepatitis B virus is found in body fluids like blood, semen, or vaginal secretions. It can be transmitted through all types of sexual intercourse—oral, anal, vaginal—as well as by kissing. It can also be spread through instruments such as needles used for IV drugs, tattooing, ear piercing, acupuncture, and medical or dental work, if they are contaminated with infected blood. Hepatitis B germs can also be contracted by using a razor, toothbrush, eating utensil, towel, or toilet facility that has come into contact with contaminated body fluids, blood, or body wastes.

Transmission can occur through direct or indirect contact with a person who has an active case of hepatitis B or through contact with a hepatitis B carrier. A carrier is a person who seems to be over the disease, but still has the virus within his or her body and can infect others.

Avoiding sexual contact with anyone who has active or inactive hepatitis B is the best way to prevent catching it. Persons with the disease must take the responsibility of telling their sex partners and refraining from sexual relations. General cleanliness—washing hands thoroughly after using the toilet, avoiding dirty toilet seats, not sharing personal items like razors or douche equipment—is also essential. Using foam and condoms during anal intercourse and washing the genitals, and particularly the anus, before and after sexual contact, are also advised as extra precautions during any sexual encounter.

People experiencing hepatitis B symptoms should consult a doctor. After the second week of infection, hepatitis B can be identified through a blood test. Since it is a viral disease, there is no cure; the disease must run its course. In the meantime, the treatment is bed rest, lots of fluids, and a light, healthy diet. There is good news for hepatitis patients: people who have had hepatitis B once do not usually get it again. Unfortunately, there is bad news as well.

- There is a 10 percent mortality rate with the disease due to a widespread destruction of liver cells (Nourse, 77).
- In addition, 30 percent of people who recover from this disease still carry active virus in their bloodstream, and, although they show no symptoms, can infect others with the hepatitis B virus (ibid.).

Venereal warts. Venereal warts are hard, wrinkled bumps that appear in the genital and rectal areas. They are caused by the human papilloma virus. They are usually painless unless irritated; then they may become itchy.

Venereal warts are transmitted by direct contact between the wart and another person's skin. This can happen through vaginal, oral, or anal intercourse. However, not everyone who comes in contact with them develops these warts. The best way to avoid warts is to refrain from sexual intercourse with someone who has them. Foam and condoms may be of some help in preventing their spread.

No tests are required to determine the existence of venereal warts; a doctor's examination is sufficient. Warts must be removed before they become enlarged and spread. They can be removed chemically with an ointment or liquid called podophyllin, frozen off with dry ice, or surgically removed under a local anesthetic.

Venereal warts may return and have to be removed again. Although the virus probably never leaves the body, it is most contagious when warts are present. Babies born of mothers with venereal warts may develop growths in or around the larynx.

BACTERIA

While some STDs are caused by viruses, others are caused by bacteria. Bacteria are microscopic organisms that can only be seen by the naked eye when they are grown in a special culture. The culture provides the right foodstuff, temperature, and climate for the bacteria to multiply by the millions, creating a colony. This colony can be seen without a microscope.

The dark, moist, warm parts of the human body provide a climate that readily supports bacteria of various types, some of which cause sexually transmitted diseases. Bacteria cannot survive very long outside such a supportive climate, so they cannot be picked up on toilet seats, doorknobs, or towels. They can be killed with antibiotics.

Gonorrhea. Gonorrhea, also called the clap or drip, is caused by gonococcus bacteria. Gonococcus is highly infectious and gonorrhea is currently the most widespread STD.

- 2.5 million cases of gonorrhea are reported per year (Neu, 443).

- In 1984, almost 20,000 cases of gonorrhea were reported among 10-to-19-year-olds (U.S. Department of Health and Human Services, 58).
- Gonorrhea is sometimes difficult to diagnose because 80 percent of the females and 20–30 percent of the males who contract it show no symptoms (Bell, 231).

A female with gonorrhea may secrete an unusual-smelling, thick, whitish, yellowish, or greenish discharge from her vagina. She may also have lower abdominal pain, painful urination, sore throat, swollen glands, and/or discharge from her anus. A male may notice a drip or discharge from his penis before his first morning urination. This drip sometimes continues throughout the day. A male may also experience burning or painful urination, sore throat, swollen glands, and/or discharge from his anus.

When these symptoms occur, it usually has been between one day and two weeks after contact with the infected areas of another person's body. Because gonorrhea germs grow in warm, dark, moist areas of the body, they thrive in the vagina, penis, throat, mouth, and anus. Thus any type of sexual intercourse—vaginal, anal, or oral—can transmit gonorrhea. The eyes can become infected too if they come in contact with the bacteria. Although symptoms may not occur or not show up for several days, the bacteria can be passed to another sex partner immediately.

Regular use of foam and condoms or diaphragms and jelly can help prevent transmission and is advised because people often are unaware they are contagious. Of course, sexual contact with a person with known gonorrhea should be avoided.

Because so many people with gonorrhea show no symptoms, sexually active teens who have more than one partner or whose partners have other partners should be tested for gonorrhea twice a year. For a male who has a discharge from his penis, the doctor may do a Gram's stain test. If there is no discharge, a culture test will be performed on cells taken from his penis, throat, or anus. The Gram's stain test is not reliable for a female, so she must have a culture taken from her cervix, anus, throat, and/or urethra, depending on the types of intercourse she has had.

Gonorrhea can be cured with penicillin, ampicillin, and tetracycline, which the doctor will prescribe as soon as the disease is diagnosed. Unfortunately, people who do not suspect they have gonorrhea cannot begin treatment, and untreated gonorrhea can have serious consequences such as permanent sterility, crippling arthritis, or blindness. Babies born to mothers with gonorrhea can go blind unless drops of nitric acid are put into their eyes. This is why routine gonorrhea tests and knowing the symptoms of gonorrhea are so important.

Chlamydia. Chlamydia is also known as NGU (nongonococcal urethritis) or NSU (nonspecific urethritis). An inflammation of the urethra, this STD is most often caused by the chlamydia trachomatis bacterium. It is a very common disease.

- "Chlamydial infection remains the most common sexually transmitted disease in the United States" (National Institute of Allergy and Infectious Diseases, 1).
- "About 5–7 million new cases of chlamydia occur each year" (ibid.).
- It is estimated that in some communities nearly one-third of the sexually active teenage girls have chlamydia (Eagan, 149).

Chlamydia's symptoms, which appear around 10 to 20 days after contact with an infected person, include discharge from the penis or cervix, painful urination, bladder infections, itchiness around the penis or vagina, or abdominal pain. However, most people have no symptoms from chlamydia, making it difficult to detect the presence of the disease, which is transmitted through oral, vaginal, or anal sexual intercourse.

Avoiding intercourse with anyone who knows he or she has chlamydia is imperative, and using condoms and spermicidal foam during vaginal or anal intercourse is advised. Chlamydia can be detected by a culture test and cured with the antibiotic tetracycline. Anyone diagnosed for chlamydia has the responsibility of notifying his or her sex partners that they need to be tested. This is often the only way people know they may be at risk.

Untreated chlamydia can lead to damage to the reproductive system, which could result in sterility. Babies born to women with chlamydia may have birth defects, eye damage, or pneumonia. Once the disease is cured, the person who had it is no longer contagious, but he or she may catch it again from an infected sex partner.

Syphilis. Syphilis, also called siff, pox, or bad blood, is an STD caused by tiny spiral treponema pallidum bacteria, which can live only inside human bodies.

- In 1984, there were almost 70,000 cases of syphilis (U.S. Department of Health and Human Services, 54).
- Of the cases reported in 1984, 25 cases occurred with 10-to-19-year-olds (ibid., 63).

One of the primary symptoms of syphilis occurs about three weeks after contact with an infected person. A hard, reddish-brown, painless sore, called a chancre (pronounced shanker) forms at the spot where the bacterium entered the body—usually around the mouth, genital, or rectal area. The chancre contains a watery liquid that is highly concentrated with bacteria. The disease is extremely contagious at this stage.

After the chancre appears, lymph glands in the groin may swell with syphilis bacteria. If an infected person is treated at this stage, the chancre and swelling will disappear and the person is cured. He or she is no longer in danger of further complications or of infecting anyone else. If the infected person is not treated, the primary symptoms will go away in three to five weeks, but the disease will remain.

In several months, the second stage of syphilis may start. Some people show no signs at this stage, but others do. Symptoms might include fever, aches, sore throat, mouth sores, patches of hair loss, swollen glands, and a general flulike feeling. A rash on the palms of the hands and the soles of the feet may also appear.

As in the primary stage, if the patient is treated at this point, he or she will be cured and free from danger of complications or transmission. If not treated, these symptoms will also disappear after a few months. The disease remains, but has now gone into a latent or hidden stage.

Months or years later (it could even be 20 to 40 years), the disease may resurface and begin to attack the heart, brain, muscles, or bones, causing spinal cord damage, brain cell destruction, heart disease, blindness, muscle incoordination, deafness, paralysis, insanity, and death.

Syphilis is transmitted in three ways: through sexual intercourse with someone who has a chancre in his or her genital or rectal region; by kissing someone with a chancre on or in his or her mouth; or through a pregnant woman's placenta to her unborn baby. Transmission can be prevented by avoiding sexual contact, even kissing, with anyone who has a syphilis chancre or a rash on his or her hands or feet. Using foam and condoms is always advised whenever there is any possibility a sex partner may have syphilis.

The unborn baby of a syphilitic mother can be born undamaged if the syphilis is discovered and treated before the sixteenth or eighteenth week of pregnancy. Otherwise, the baby will probably be born dead.

Discovering syphilis requires a blood test called a VDRL. Every pregnant girl should have one of these done as soon as she learns she is pregnant. The treatment for syphilis is a time-released injection of penicillin or some other antibiotic. This will cure the disease at whatever stage it has progressed to, but it cannot repair any damage to the body that has already occurred.

Yeast infections. A certain amount of yeast and bacteria normally grow in a girl's vagina. The bacteria generally keep the multiplication of yeast organisms under control, but sometimes the yeast gets out of control and a yeast infection occurs. If this happens, a thick, white, curdlike vaginal discharge will appear. Genitals (female or male) with a yeast infection are usually red, itchy, and smell like yeast. Although yeast infections are unpleasant, they are not dangerous unless the girl is pregnant.

Yeast infections may be caused by the use of antibiotics that upset the bacterial balance of the vagina. They may also be caused by taking birth-control pills. Yeast infections can be transmitted to sexual partners through oral, vaginal, or anal intercourse. Babies born to mothers with a yeast infection may pick up the disease as they pass through the birth canal and develop a yeast infection in their mouths called thrush.

Keeping the genital area clean, avoiding perfumed products in the genital area, not wearing tight pants, limiting sugar intake, using plain white toilet paper, and using barrier protection (condom or diaphragm) and a spermicidal foam or cream during intercourse can help protect against the spread of yeast infections. Girls using the birth-control pill may want to consider another form of contraception.

Doctors test for yeast infections by placing a sample of the discharge on a slide and examining it under the microscope. The treatment for yeast infection is a prescription drug called Mycostatin or some other form of nystatin.

PARASITES

In addition to bacteria and viruses, another way STDs are spread is through parasites. Parasites are tiny, one-celled organisms that live on or in the human body and depend on it for their food. There are many such organisms on or in human bodies, and some of these are passed from person to person during sexual activities. Because these organisms can survive outside the body for varying lengths of time, they can also be picked up from inanimate objects such as infected towels, clothes, or personal articles.

Trichomonas vaginalis. Trichomonas vaginalis or trichomoniasis, commonly called trich (pronounced "trick"), in girls is a vaginal infection caused by a trichomonas vaginalis organism. In boys, it is developed in the prostate gland.

Symptoms for girls include a thin, yellow-green or milky-gray, foul-smelling vaginal discharge accompanied by itching and a burning sensation during urination. Boys will experience a discharge from the penis and a tickling during urination.

Trich is transmitted by any sort of sexual contact including touching of genitals as well as all types of sexual intercourse. It can be passed through the semen of an infected boy.

Because the parasite can stay alive for up to seven hours outside the body, it can be passed by using someone else's washcloth or towel or wearing another person's bathing suit or unclean underwear. It can even be picked up on an infected toilet seat.

Refraining from sexual contact and not sharing personal items until the infection is cured can help prevent its spread. Vinegar-water douches for girls, especially during menstruation, can also be effective.

Testing for trich involves a health professional examining a sample of the discharge on a slide under a microscope. A drug named Flagyl is the only treatment available, but it is dangerous, particularly for pregnant girls, and should not be taken without consulting a doctor.

Pubic lice. Pubic lice or crab lice, or crabs as they are commonly called, are pinhead-sized yellowish-gray animals that feed on human blood. They thrive in moist, hairy spots, such as pubic, underarm, or chest hair and even eyelashes. They lay their eggs, nits, at these sites as well.

Itchiness is the main symptom of crabs because when they bite, crabs inject human blood with a chemical that causes intense itching. The waste matter they give off also causes itchiness. They sometimes carry diseases such as typhus.

Crabs are highly contagious and can jump from one person to another. Sexual intercourse is a prime time for their transmission. Crabs can survive for about 24 hours without a source of blood and their eggs can survive away from a moist, hairy spot for about a week. This, and their jumping ability, mean that they can be picked up almost anywhere. However, sharing bedding, clothing, and personal items with someone infested with crabs is especially risky.

Avoiding contact with anyone who has crabs and keeping oneself and one's linens, clothing, and personal items clean are the best ways to prevent the spread of crabs.

Crabs can be seen with the naked eye, so there is no test necessary for their diagnosis. Soap and water will not kill them, but a prescription cream called Kwell is effective against them. Clothing and bedding must be washed in hot water with a detergent or dry-cleaned.

Scabies. Scabies mites are smaller than crabs and burrow under one's skin to lay their eggs. They give off waste products in their under-the-skin burrows, which cause considerable itching. Other symptoms include skin infections in the areas between the fingers, on the elbows, in the armpits, on the breasts, in the genital region, and on the buttocks. These infections are blisterlike sores or raised reddish tracks.

Highly contagious, scabies are transmitted through any kind of touching, whether casual or intimate. They can also be spread via bed sheets or clothing infected with the scabies mites or their eggs. To prevent their transmission, avoid physical contact, especially sexual contact, with any infected person or his or her clothing or bedding. Personal hygiene is essential.

Scabies can be diagnosed by examining some of the skin scrapings under a microscope. The treatment, Kwell cream as prescribed by a doctor, is the same as for crabs.

Conclusion

Although some STDs are primarily an inconvenient irritation that can be fairly easily cured, others are much more serious. The potential for lifelong problems and even death demands responsible decisions about sexual activities.

REFERENCES

Bell, Ruth, et al. *Changing Bodies, Changing Lives: A Book for Teens on Sex and Relationships.* New York: Random House, 1987.

Busch, Phyllis S. *What about VD?* New York: Four Winds Press, 1976.

Centers for Disease Control, Center for Health Promotion and Education. *Morbidity and Mortality Weekly Report: Guidelines for Effective School Health Education To Prevent the Spread of AIDS.* Vol. 37. Atlanta: U.S. Department of Health and Human Services, January 29, 1988.

Eagan, Andrea Boroff. *Why Am I So Miserable If These Are the Best Years of My Life?: Everything Your Mother Never Told You about Becoming a Woman.* New York: Avon, 1988.

Hein, Karen, M.D., and Theresa Foy DiGeronimo. *AIDS: Trading Fears for Facts: A Guide for Teens.* Mount Vernon, NY: Consumers Union, 1989.

Kurland, Morton L., M.D. *Coping with AIDS: Facts and Fears.* New York: Rosen Publishing Co., 1987.

Langone, John. *AIDS: The Facts.* New York: Little, Brown, 1988.

Madaras, Lynda. *Lynda Madaras Talks to Teens about AIDS: An Essential Guide for Parents, Teachers, and Young People.* New York: Newmarket, 1988.

National Institute of Allergy and Infectious Diseases. *Sexually Transmitted Diseases, 1987 Research Report.* Washington, DC: Office of Communications, January 1988.

Neu, Harold C., M.D. "Infectious Diseases." In *The Columbia University College of Physicians and Surgeons Complete Home Medical Guide,* ed. Donald F. Tapley, M.D., et al., 425–451. Mount Vernon, NY: Consumers Union, 1985.

Nourse, Alan E., M.D. *Herpes.* New York: Franklin Watts, 1985.

Ulene, Art, M.D. *Safe Sex in a Dangerous World: Understanding and Coping with the Threat of AIDS.* New York: Vintage, 1987.

U.S. Department of Health and Human Services, Public Health Service, Centers for Disease Control, Center for Prevention Services, Division of Sexually Transmitted Diseases. *Sexually Transmitted Disease Statistics 1984.* Atlanta: U.S. Government Printing Office, 1985.

Resources
for Finding Out about Sexually Transmitted Diseases

Sexually Transmitted Diseases in Fiction

Sexually transmitted diseases provide the focus for some of these young-adult novels; in others, STDs are merely mentioned. The recent AIDS epidemic has encouraged authors to write books on this important topic.

Blume, Judy. **Forever.** Scarsdale, NY: Bradbury (Pocket Books), 1975. 220p.

In this classic book about teenage sexuality, Katherine and Michael start going together as high school seniors. Michael is more sexually experienced than Katherine. He has had intercourse twice with a casual acquaintance from whom he contracted VD. He assures Katherine he is cured, and they decide they would like to have sex.

Dizenzo, Patricia. **Why Me? The Story of Jenny.** New York: Avon, 1976. 142p.

Fifteen-year-old Jenny is raped by a stranger from whom she accepted a ride on a very cold night. She cannot tell her parents for fear that they will not believe her. She only tells one friend, who does not seem to be of any help to her. All alone, she copes with a visit to a clinic and the system of venereal-disease tests.

Hermes, Patricia. **Be Still My Heart.** New York: Putnam's, 1989. 144p.

Allison and David are selected as editors of their school yearbook. They soon learn that the husband of their yearbook advisor, Ms. Adams, has been diagnosed as having AIDS. The students in the high school do not know exactly what AIDS is, but they know people with AIDS die. Upset at the discrimination Ms. Adams is forced to face because of her husband, Allison sets out on a campaign to inform the school about the realities of AIDS and its victims. Through her efforts, Allison learns to stand up for what she believes.

Kerr, M. E. **Night Kites.** New York: Harper & Row (Harper Keypoint), 1986. 216p.
High school senior Erick Rudd can't believe how lucky he is to be having a passionate love affair with the exotic Nicki. Not only is Nicki helping him explore his sexuality, she is also helping take his mind off his home situation. The Rudd family is in an uproar because Pete, Erick's older brother, has announced he has AIDS, and the family didn't even know he was gay. Through Nicki and Pete, Erick learns about being different and not fitting in. He, and the reader, learn about AIDS and the gay community as well.

Koertge, Ron. **The Arizona Kid.** Boston: Little, Brown, 1988. 228p.
Billy leaves his family and friends in Bradyville, Missouri, and spends the summer in Arizona, living with Wes, his homosexual uncle. Billy learns about love and horse tracks, but he also gains insight into the gay lifestyle of his uncle and the gay community's concern about AIDS. Wes has friends who have died from AIDS, and he works on an AIDS hotline. He teaches Billy the importance of practicing safe sex.

Levy, Marilyn. **Putting Heather Together Again.** New York: Ballantine (Fawcett Juniper), 1989. 136p.
After 17-year-old Heather is raped, she has a gynecological exam in which she is tested for STDs.

Miklowitz, Gloria D. **Good-bye Tomorrow.** New York: Delacorte (Dell), 1987. 150p.

Senior Alex Weiss is infected with the AIDS virus during a blood transfusion. Alex, who once had everything going for him, now has ARC (AIDS-related complex) and his whole life changes. In this well-researched novel, Alex, his sister Christi, and his girlfriend Shannon each present his/her own version of what happened to Alex and how each of them deals with the situation.

Nonfiction Materials on Sexually Transmitted Diseases

The works listed below represent a variety of resources on sexually transmitted diseases. The comprehensive handbooks contain information about the various types of STDs. Some of the other works are concerned with a specific disease. Due to the recent need for information about AIDS, a number of books about AIDS have been added to the literature on STDs. A cross section of these is included here.

BOOKS

Alyson, Sasha, ed. **You Can Do Something about AIDS.** Boston: Stop AIDS Project, 1988. 126p.

This collection of short essays by famous or authoritative people suggests what various individuals, professions, and organizations can do about AIDS. The book was produced as a public service project of the publishing industry and is free of charge.

Bell, Ruth, et al. **Changing Bodies, Changing Lives: A Book for Teens on Sex and Relationships.** New York: Random House (Vintage Books), 1987. 254p.

This comprehensive book, written specifically for teenagers, includes information on all aspects of teen sexuality and general health. In a section called "Sexually Transmitted Diseases and How To Avoid Them," the authors describe the various STDs and their treatments. AIDS is included in this updated version of this excellent resource for teens.

Eagan, Andrea Boroff. **Why Am I So Miserable If These Are the Best Years of My Life?: Everything Your Mother Never Told You about Becoming a Woman.** New York: Avon, 1988. 211p.

Eagan's background in the women's health movement is evident as she explains the causes, symptoms, and cures (where they exist) for the various STDs. Her information is factual and her style straightforward and interesting.

Gulas, Ivan, and Leslie Griffiths. **Herpes: The Love Bug: Facts and Fears.** Columbus: Ohio Psychology Publishing, 1984. 59p.

The first part of this very readable little book describes the physical aspects of herpes, and the second part discusses the psychological aspects involved in acquiring herpes.

Hawkes, Nigel. **AIDS.** New York: Gloucester, 1987. 32p.

Using color photographs, diagrams, and a straightforward text, this book provides an international perspective. Facts and figures about AIDS around the world are provided. This short, compelling book would be appropriate for young adolescents.

Hyde, Margaret O., and Elizabeth H. Forsyth, M.D. **AIDS: What Does It Mean to You?** New York: Walker, 1987. 116p.

Written for an adolescent audience, this book presents information about the causes of AIDS, what it is like to have AIDS, ways to prevent the spread of AIDS, and the effect AIDS could have on the future. Information about past epidemics adds a historical perspective. The complete "Surgeon General's Report on Acquired Immune Deficiency Syndrome," a short list of groups offering AIDS information and support, a glossary, and an index are also included.

Jacobs, George, and Joseph Kerins, M.D. **What We Need To Know about AIDS Now!: The AIDS File.** Woods Hole, MA: Cromlech, 1987. 128p.

The authors present fairly detailed information about AIDS and related topics. Technical material is clearly explained. A glossary and index are included.

Johnson, Eric W. **Love & Sex in Plain Language.** Philadelphia: Lippincott (Bantam), 1985. 207p.

Along with other topics concerning sex and sexuality, the author discusses sexually transmitted diseases including AIDS. This book is not difficult to read. Illustrations, glossary, and index make the information readily accessible. Originally written in 1968, this is the fourth revision of this concise but comprehensive book.

Krumkin, Lyn, M.D., and John Leonard, M.D. **Questions & Answers on AIDS.** New York: Avon, 1987. 203p.

Using a question and answer format, the authors explain what the AIDS virus is, how it attacks, risk factors involved, and the latest medical advances. A list of AIDS resource centers and a glossary are included.

Kuklin, Susan. **Fighting Back: What Some People Are Doing about AIDS.** New York: Putnam's, 1989. 110p.

This book describes the work of the Gay Men's Health Crisis, Inc. (GMHC), a group dedicated to supporting people with AIDS (PWAs). Volunteers, both homosexual and heterosexual, help PWAs in ways such as doing domestic chores and listening to them talk about the disease. Through the stories of the PWAs and the volunteers, the reader comes to understand something of the disease and what it is like to have it. The reader also comes to appreciate the efforts of the GMHC and religious groups like the Catholic Church. A glossary is included.

Kurland, Morton L., M.D. **Coping with AIDS: Facts and Fears.** New York: Rosen Publishing Group, 1987. 118p.

The author explains the theory that AIDS started in Africa with the green monkeys and spread through the rest of the world. He describes what the AIDS virus does to human beings and how it is transmitted. Case studies of AIDS patients, most of whom are interviewed by a therapist, illustrate how they contracted AIDS and their reactions to the diagnosis. Kurland writes factually and uses analogies for clarification. The book is appropriate for more mature adolescents. An appendix includes lists of AIDS crisis centers throughout the world.

Langone, John. **AIDS: The Facts.** Boston: Little, Brown, 1988. 247p.

This thorough and technical, but readable, coverage of AIDS information is an excellent reference for older adolescents or adults wanting a scholarly approach to the subject.

Lingle, Virginia A., and M. Sandra Woods. **How To Find Information about AIDS.** New York: Harrington Park Press, 1988. 130p.

This book provides comprehensive lists of organizational resources, health departments, research institutions, grant-funding sources, federal agencies, hotlines, computerized and print sources of information, and audiovisual producers throughout the United States that are concerned with AIDS. It is well organized, and a general index and geographic index make it easy to use.

Madaras, Lynda. **Lynda Madaras Talks to Teens about AIDS: An Essential Guide for Parents, Teachers, and Young People.** New York: Newmarket, 1988. 160p.

The purpose of this book is to help 14-to-19-year-olds understand the facts about AIDS and its prevention. The information provided is comprehensive and well researched. Madaras writes in a frank manner, defining and explaining important terms as necessary. She clarifies the facts about AIDS and provides specific guidelines for preventing its transmission. She includes information about contraceptives that can help prevent the spread of AIDS, along with an index and a list of sources for further information. This book is an excellent resource.

Madaras, Lynda, with Area Madaras. **The What's Happening to My Body? Book for Girls: A Growing Up Guide for Parents and Daughters.** New York: Newmarket, 1988. 269p.

This book was written especially for younger adolescents and their parents by a sex educator and her teenage daughter. Although the primary focus is female puberty, the authors include information on the types, symptoms, spread, and prevention of STDs and testing for them. The frank, clear explanations and conversational writing style make information accessible to the intended audience. Illustrations enhance the text, and an index is included.

Madaras, Lynda, with Dane Saavedra. **The What's Happening to My Body? Book for Boys: A Growing Up Guide for Parents and Sons.** New York: Newmarket, 1987. 251p.

Written by a sex educator with the assistance of a teenage boy, the primary topic of this book is male puberty. The authors also present information on STDs, including descriptions of the various diseases, their symptoms, how they are spread, how they are tested, and how to prevent their transmission. The intended audience is younger adolescents and their parents. This book is highly useful and informative, and the conversational style makes the information accessible to teens. An index and illustrations are included.

Masters, William H., M.D., Virginia E. Johnson, and Robert C. Kolodny, M.D. **Crisis: Heterosexual Behavior in the Age of AIDS.** New York: Grove Press, 1988. 243p.

Written by well-known medical researchers in the field of human sexuality, this book provides in-depth information about AIDS and stresses the seriousness of the problem. The question of safe sex is discussed in detail. The authors believe that large numbers of adolescents engage in high-risk behaviors for acquiring AIDS, and that these behaviors must change if the AIDS epidemic is to be curbed. This is a useful reference book for older adolescents and adults working with young adults.

McCoy, Kathy, and Charles Wibbelsman, M.D. **The New Teenage Body Book.** Los Angeles: Body Press, 1987. 278p.

Concerned with the overall health of teenagers, this handbook contains a section on sexually transmitted diseases. Names and addresses of nationwide agencies that can help teenagers with health and sexual concerns are provided in the appendix. Illustrations and an index are also included. Readable and comprehensive, this handbook is an excellent resource for teenagers.

Nourse, Alan E., M.D. **Herpes.** New York: Franklin Watts, 1985. 104p.

Appropriately detailed information about the herpes virus and the rapidly increasing spread of this sexually transmitted disease is provided for an adolescent audience. Information about prevention and treatment is included. Other STDs are described, as is the current state of herpes research, in this informative and readable book. An index is included.

Surgeon General's Report on Acquired Immune Deficiency Syndrome. Washington, DC: U.S. Department of Health and Human Services, 1986. 36p.

C. Everett Koop, M.D., Sc.D., former surgeon general for the U.S. Public Health Service, provides basic information about transmission, risk of infection, and prevention of AIDS. Koop's message is straightforward and factual. He dispels common misconceptions about the disease and stresses that AIDS can and must be stopped. He includes a list of telephone hotlines and national sources of information.

Ulene, Art, M.D. **Safe Sex in a Dangerous World: Understanding and Coping with the Threat of AIDS.** New York: Vintage, 1987. 109p.

The Family Doctor from the "Today" show discusses AIDS and how to prevent its spread. In this frank, easy-to-read little book, he emphasizes safe sex and explains the risks involved with different types of sex partners and different types of sex.

Wachter, Oralee. **Sex, Drugs & AIDS.** New York: Bantam, 1987. 76p.

Based on a film with the same title, this short book presents the basic facts about AIDS. The message is clear and direct:

avoid the risk of AIDS by not sharing needles and by using condoms during sexual intercourse. There are black and white photographs of actress Rae Dawn Chong, who narrates the film, and of people who have AIDS and who explain how the disease is transmitted. A question and answer section addresses questions commonly asked about AIDS.

Weston, Carol. **Girltalk about Guys.** New York: Harper & Row, 1988. 220p.

Although Weston devotes two-thirds of this book to the topics of attraction to the opposite sex, dating, and breaking up, she also includes a section on protecting oneself from STDs. She describes the various types of STDs, including AIDS. The author's chatty style makes the information easy to read and her advice easy to consider.

Young, Proud and Gay! Boston: Alyson, 1985. 94p.

Written specifically for gay and lesbian teenagers by gays and lesbians, this book provides detailed information about gay sexuality. The chapter entitled "Gays and Health" includes an excellent section about symptoms of and treatments for STDs, including AIDS. Illustrations and annotated bibliographies enhance the text. The writing is straightforward and informative.

ARTICLES

"Can You Rely on Condoms?" *Consumer Reports* (March 1989): 135–141.

The research staff of *Consumer Reports* tested various brands of condoms for their effectiveness against breakage. They also surveyed 3,300 readers about their use of condoms and knowledge about AIDS. Detailed reports of this research are given in this article.

"Questions about AIDS," *Consumer Reports* (March 1989): 142.

Answers are given to commonly asked questions about AIDS.

Nonprint Materials on Sexually Transmitted Diseases

A sampling of films and videocassettes about sexually transmitted diseases is listed. Due to the recent demand for information about AIDS, most of the items listed are about this topic. Reviewing sources included *School Library Booklist, Video Source Book, Lander's Film Review,* and *Media Review Digest.*

AIDS
Type:	16mm film, VHS videocassette
Length:	19 min.
Cost:	Rental $65; purchase $455 (film), $345 (video)
Distributor:	Walt Disney Educational Media Co.
	Coronet MTI Film and Video
	108 W. Wilmot Road
	Deerfield, IL 60615
Date:	1987

Narrated by actress Ally Sheedy, this film on AIDS is aimed at junior and senior high school students.

AIDS: Answers for Young People
Type:	Videocassette
Length:	18 min.
Distributor:	Boulton-Hawker Films
	Hadleigh, Ipswitch
	Suffolk, England 1P7 5BG
Date:	1987

This videotape, designed for teenagers, explains how to prevent getting and giving AIDS.

AIDS: Changing the Rules
Type:	VHS videocassette
Length:	27 min.
Cost:	Purchase $44.95
Distributor:	AIDSFILMS
	50 W. 34th Street, Suite 6B6
	New York, NY 10001
Date:	1987

Information on AIDS transmission and prevention is supplied in this film.

AIDS: Facts and Fears, Crisis and Controversy
Type: VHS videocassette
Length: 56 min.
Cost: Purchase $209
Distributor: Guidance Associates, Inc.
Communications Park, Box 3000
Mt. Kisco, NY 10549
Date: 1986

Medical experts explain the clinical nature of the virus and how it attacks the body. The scope of the epidemic is discussed and high-risk behaviors are identified.

AIDS: Facts over Fear
Type: 16mm film, videocassette
Length: 10 min.
Cost: Rental $65; purchase $250 (film), $200 (video)
Distributor: Coronet MTI Film and Video
108 Wilmot Road
Deerfield, IL 60015
Date: 1985

This ABC "20-20" production, hosted by Barbara Walters, is an investigative report that looks beyond the hysteria surrounding the disease and focuses on the facts provided by current medical research.

AIDS: One Family's Story
Type: VHS videocassette
Length: 36 min.
Cost: Rental $75; purchase $185
Distributor: Sunburst Communications
Room RB36
101 Castleton Street
Pleasantville, NY 10570-3498
Date: 1988

Ryan, 18, learns his father is gay and is dying of AIDS.

AIDS Alert for Youth
Type: VHS videocassette
Length: 13 min.
Cost: Rental $55; purchase $115
Distributor: Sunburst Communications
Room RB36
101 Castleton Street
Pleasantville, NY 10570-3498
Date: 1989

A question and answer format provides the correct medical facts about AIDS. This video is designed for students in grades 5–9. Dr. Richard Keeling, a leading authority on AIDS, is featured at the beginning of the tape.

The AIDS Epidemic: Is *Anyone* Safe?
Type: VHS videocassette
Length: 50 min.
Cost: Purchase $175
Distributor: Guidance Associates, Inc.
Communications Park, Box 3000
Mt. Kisco, NY 10549
Date: 1987

Interviews with medical experts give teens information on how to protect themselves by abstaining from sex, using condoms, or avoiding certain types of activities. Common myths about how AIDS is transmitted are examined and dispelled.

AIDS Hits Home
Type: VHS videocassette
Length: 48 min.
Cost: Rental $45; purchase $330
Distributor: Carousel Film and Video
260 Fifth Avenue, Room 705
New York, NY 10001
Date: 1986

This television news special features interviews, comments, and statistics detailing the known history of AIDS and how it spreads.

AIDS in Your School
Type: Videocassette
Length: 23 min.
Cost: Purchase $164
Distributor: Peregrine Productions
c/o Perennial Education
930 Pitner Avenue
Evanston, IL 60202
Date: 1987

In this program designed for high school students, the causes and effects of AIDS are outlined through interviews of a physician and several AIDS patients.

The Best Defense
Type: VHS videocassette
Length: 20 min.
Cost: $229
Distributor: Intermedia
1300 Dexter North
Seattle, WA 98109
Date: 1988

The first part of this video focuses on educating intravenous drug users about bleaching needles in an effort to protect themselves aginst the AIDS virus. The second part portrays a couple discussing safe sex, and the final section depicts a Latino couple wrestling with the early signs of infection by the AIDS virus. The message is that AIDS can be spread by sharing needles or having unprotected sex with someone who has shared needles. Available in both English and Spanish.

Choices
Type: VHS videocassette
Length: 20 min.
Cost: Purchase $189
Distributor: Intermedia
1300 Dexter North
Seattle, WA 98109
Date: 1988

A group of friends discovers that the brother of one of their members has AIDS, and they must deal with the reality of the disease and their feelings about it. Through their conversation, viewers learn about the facts, misconceptions, common fears, and practical choices regarding AIDS.

Close Encounters of the Sexual Kind
Type: Videocassette
Length: 12 min.
Cost: Purchase $125
Distributor: Filmakers Library
124 E. 40th Street
New York, NY 10016
Date: 1989

Information about several sexually transmitted diseases and the social attitudes toward them are explored. The video promotes the practice of safe sex by using condoms during sexual intercourse.

Coping with Herpes Series: A Family of Viruses
Type: VHS videocassette
Length: 14 min.
Cost: Rental $35; purchase $235
Distributor: Perennial Education, Inc.
930 Pitner Avenue
Evanston, IL 60202
Date: 1988

This introductory program discusses the five types of herpes and how the most widely known types—oral and genital—are contracted.

Coping with Herpes Series: Herpes and Long-Term Relationships
Type: VHS videocassette
Length: 11 min.
Cost: Rental $35; purchase $235
Distributor: Perennial Education, Inc.
930 Pitner Avenue
Evanston, IL 60202
Date: 1988

This program discusses the challenge of coping with herpes within a long-term relationship.

Coping with Herpes Series: Herpes and Pregnancy
Type: VHS videocassette
Length: 8 min.
Cost: Rental $35; purchase $235
Distributor: Perennial Education, Inc.
930 Pitner Avenue
Evanston, IL 60202
Date: 1988

This program explores the necessary precautions, medical tests, and the possibility of cesarean delivery when a pregnant woman has herpes.

Coping with Herpes Series: Herpes and Single People
Type: VHS videocassette
Length: 10 min.
Cost: Rental $35; purchase $235
Distributor: Perennial Education, Inc.
930 Pitner Avenue
Evanston, IL 60202
Date: 1988

This program helps herpes sufferers put the disease into perspective.

Coping with Herpes Series: Treatment and Management of Symptoms
Type: VHS videocassette
Length: 12 min.
Cost: Rental $35; purchase $235
Distributor: Perennial Education, Inc.
930 Pitner Avenue
Evanston, IL 60202
Date: 1988

Herpes researcher Dr. Yvonne Bryson discusses some of the ways to manage and treat herpes symptoms.

Don't Forget Sherri
Type: VHS or Beta videocassette
Length: 30 min.
Distributor: American Red Cross
c/o Millie Burns
1709 New York Avenue NW, Suite 208
Washington, DC 20006
Date: 1987

This love story, which investigates the budding relationship between two urban teenagers who are questioning their own personal values and behavior, provides an opportunity for teens to view the impact of the spread of the AIDS virus through the eyes of teens like themselves.

"Herpie": The New VD around Town (rev. ed.)
Type: VHS or Beta videocassette
Length: 15 min.
Cost: Rental $55; purchase $95
Distributor: International Film Bureau
332 South Michigan Avenue, Suite 522
Chicago, IL 60604
Date: 1988

Cartoon character Herpie talks about prevention of herpes, and, for those already infected, how to minimize transmission and effects.

Mi Hermano
Type: VHS videocassette
Length: 28 min.
Distributor: American Red Cross
c/o Dr. Rebeca Gilad, Director
Hispanic AIDS Education Program
1709 New York Avenue NW, Suite 208
Washington DC, 20006
Date: 1990

This film centers around a Hispanic immigrant family that has lost a son to AIDS. Basic AIDS information is conveyed as family members try to learn how the young man contracted the disease. This video is available both in Spanish and in Spanish with English subtitles.

Sex, Drugs, & AIDS
Type: 16mm film, VHS videocassette
Length: 18 min.
Cost: Rental $75; purchase $400 (film), $325 (video)
Distributor: Select Media, Inc.
74 Varick Street
Suite 304
New York, NY 10013
Date: 1987

This film, hosted by actress Rae Dawn Chong, is designed for teenage audiences. A book of the same title is based on the film.

Sexually Transmitted Diseases
Type: Videocassette
Length: 20 min.
Distributor: Medfact Inc.
P.O. Box 418
Massillon, OH 44648
Date: 1986

A video designed to teach the average person the basics of venereal disease transmission, symptoms, and prevention.

Sexually Transmitted Diseases: What You Should Know
Type: 35mm film, VHS videocassette
Length: 27 min.
Cost: Rental $75; purchase $129 (film), $165 (video)
Distributor: Sunburst Communications
Room RB36
101 Castleton Street
Pleasantville, NY 10570-3498
Date: 1989

The focus is sexually transmitted diseases other than AIDS. The film teaches students how to be aware of these diseases and to protect themselves.

Smart Talk
Type: VHS videocassette
Length: 13 min.
Cost: Purchase $189
Distributor: Intermedia
1300 Dexter North
Seattle, WA 98109
Date: 1988

This video dispels common myths about STDs, including AIDS, and emphasizes knowing about and promptly treating all STDs.

STD Blues
Type: 16mm film, VHS videocassette
Length: 33 min.
Cost: Rental $80; purchase $595 (film), $340 (video)
Distributor: Phoenix Films/BFA Films and Video
468 Park Avenue South
New York, NY 10016
Date: 1987

The danger of contracting STDs by engaging in sexual intercourse without the use of condoms is stressed.

The STD Gang: Prevention and Treatment
Type: Videocassette
Length: 25 min.
Cost: Rental $55; purchase $129
Distributor: Sunburst Communications
Room RB36
101 Castleton Street
Pleasantville, NY 10570-3498

Five sexually transmitted diseases—gonorrhea, syphilis, nongonococcal urethritis, herpes, and trichomoniasis—are featured, with information about the symptoms, treatment, transmission, and prevention of each.

The Subject Is AIDS
Type: VHS videocassette
Length: 18 min.

176 SEXUALLY TRANSMITTED DISEASES

Cost: Rental $75; purchase $325
Distributor: Select Media, Inc.
74 Varick Street
Suite 303
New York, NY 10013
Date: 1987

Abstinence from sex is emphasized in this film for junior high school students.

Understanding AIDS: What Teens Need To Know
Type: VHS videocassette
Length: 19 min.
Cost: Rental $55; purchase $145
Distributor: Sunburst Communications
Room RB36
101 Castleton Street
Pleasantville, NY 10570-3498
Date: 1988

Experts in the field of AIDS research answer questions asked by teenagers.

A Very Delicate Matter
Type: 16mm film, VHS videocassette
Length: 30 min. or 46 min.
Cost: Rental $75; purchase $500 or $750 (film), $500 (video, either version)
Distributor: Coronet/MTI Film and Video
108 Wilmot Road
Deerfield, IL 60015
Date: 1982

This film uses a dramatic setting to tell a story about the causes and effects of acquiring gonorrhea.

What You Don't Know CAN Kill You: Sexually Transmitted Diseases and AIDS
Type: VHS videocassette
Length: 30 min.
Cost: Purchase $209

Distributor: Guidance Associates, Inc.
Communications Park, Box 3000
Mt. Kisco, NY 10549
Date: 1990

This program helps teens to become aware of the symptoms and serious health problems related to the following STDs: AIDS, genital herpes, genital warts, gonorrhea, chlamydia, syphilis, trichomoniasis, pubic lice, and candidiasis.

Organizations Concerned with Sexually Transmitted Diseases

American Social Health Association
P.O. Box 13827
Research Triangle Park, NC 27009
(919) 361-2742
Executive Director: Peggy Clark

This 75-year-old nonprofit organization sponsors hotlines for AIDS, STDs, and herpes as well as for organizations like the Herpes Resource Center.

PUBLICATIONS: Booklets on AIDS, STDs, and herpes.

Centers for Disease Control
1600 Clifton Road NE
Atlanta, GA 30333

Many of the statistics quoted publicly about AIDS and other STDs originate with this federal agency. Personnel will send written information about these topics upon request.

The Herpes Resource Center
P.O. Box 13827
Research Triangle Park, NC 27009
(919) 361-2742
Educational Program Director: Marcus Copelan

The Herpes Resource Center is part of the American Social Health Association. Its purpose is to support research and disseminate information about herpes as well as to offer human support in a calm, caring, and concerned way. This organization coordinates a network of more than 90 self-help groups throughout the country. These groups help people suffering from herpes deal with the disease's physical and social impact. Some of these groups are geared specifically to teens. Write or call for information about local support groups.

PUBLICATIONS: *Helper* (quarterly journal); printed materials on stress management; videotapes and audiotapes.

U.S. Public Health Service Public Affairs Office
Hubert H. Humphrey Building
Room 725-H
200 Independence Avenue SW
Washington, DC 20201
(202) 245-6867

PUBLICATIONS: Various pamphlets on public health concerns, including AIDS, such as the *Surgeon General's Report on Acquired Immune Deficiency Syndrome*, which is available in English and Spanish versions free of charge.

Hotlines

NATIONAL

These numbers can be reached from all over the country. Those with an 800 prefix are free of charge, and the call will not show up on your telephone bill in any form. You will need to dial a "1" before the number.

AIDS Hotline for Teens   (800) 234-TEEN
This hotline is staffed by trained high school students from 4:00 to 8:00 P.M. on Monday through Friday.

Herpes Hotline   (919) 361-2120
Experts on herpes are available for consultation and referrals from 9:00 A.M. to 6:00 P.M. Eastern Standard Time.

National AIDS Hotline   (800) 342-AIDS

You may call this number 24 hours a day and talk to someone. It is maintained by the Centers for Disease Control (CDC), and operators will provide basic information, referrals, and send written information appropriate for teens. They will also provide a telephone number so you can have access to recordings from the CDC.

National AIDS Hotline (in Spanish)   (800) 344-SIDA

This hotline is staffed 8:00 A.M. to 2:00 P.M. Eastern Standard Time Monday through Friday. A recorded message will play at other times.

National AIDS Hotline (TTY/TDD)   (800) 243-7889

This hotline is for the hearing-impaired. It is staffed from 10:00 A.M. to 10:00 P.M. Eastern Standard Time from Monday through Friday.

National Sexually Transmitted Disease Hotline, American Social Health Association   (800) 227-8922

This hotline is staffed from 8:00 A.M. to 11:00 P.M. Eastern Standard Time from Monday through Friday. At other times, a recording will supply general information about STDs. When operators are on duty, they will provide referrals to clinics, and answer questions about how to recognize and prevent STDs.

STATE

The following numbers are state AIDS hotlines. The 800 numbers are toll free in that state, territory, or district.

Alabama	(800) 228-0469 or (800) 445-3741
Alaska	(800) 478-2437
Arizona	(800) 342-2437 or (800) 334-1540
Arkansas	(800) 445-7720
California (Northern)	(800) 367-2437
California (Southern)	(800) 922-2437

180 SEXUALLY TRANSMITTED DISEASES

Colorado	(800) 252-2437
Connecticut	(800) 342-2437 or (203) 566-1157
Delaware	(800) 422-0429 or (243) 302-2437
District of Columbia	(202) 332-2437
Florida	(800) 352-2437
Georgia	(800) 551-2728
Hawaii	(808) 922-1313
Idaho	(208) 345-2277
Illinois	(800) 243-2437
Indiana	(800) 848-2437
Iowa	(800) 532-3301
Kansas	(800) 232-0040
Kentucky	(800) 654-2437
Louisiana	(800) 992-4379
Maine	(800) 851-2437
Maryland	(800) 638-6252
Massachusetts	(800) 235-2331
Michigan	(800) 872-2437
Minnesota	(800) 248-2437
Mississippi	(800) 826-2961
Missouri	(800) 533-2437
Montana	(800) 537-6187
Nebraska	(800) 782-2437
Nevada	(800) 842-2437
New Hampshire	(800) 872-8909
New Jersey	(800) 624-2377
New Mexico	(800) 545-2437
New York	(800) 541-2437
North Carolina	(800) 535-2437
North Dakota	(800) 472-2180
Ohio	(800) 332-2437
Oklahoma	(800) 522-9054
Oregon	(800) 777-2437
Pennsylvania	(800) 692-7254
Puerto Rico	(809) 765-1010 (will accept collect calls)
Rhode Island	(800) 726-3010
South Carolina	(800) 322-2437
South Dakota	(800) 592-1861
Tennessee	(800) 525-2437

Texas	(800) 248-1091
Utah	(800) 537-1046
Vermont	(800) 882-2437
Virgin Islands	(809) 773-1311
Virginia	(800) 533-4148
Washington	(800) 272-2437
West Virginia	(800) 642-8244
Wisconsin	(800) 334-2437
Wyoming	(800) 327-3577

CHAPTER 6

Unwanted Sexual Contact

He put the gun on a rock out of reach and began to take off his pants.

Like a robot, like someone in a dream, I did as he said. But I was trembling so that my fingers wouldn't undo the button on my jeans. "Don't do this to me.... I've never.... Don't! Not that!" I begged.

He whopped me again on the side of the head and shoved me to the ground. I cried out as a sharp rock cut into my hip. And then, he came down on top of me.

Gloria D. Miklowitz, *Did You Hear What Happened to Andrea?* (New York: Delacorte, 1978), 24.

"He pushed himself inside of me. He—he forced me—to have—sex with him," Heather whispered, barely able to breathe.

"He raped you."

"No," Heather replied, jumping up from her chair. "I told you, I know him. It wasn't rape."

"Did you tell him not to?"

"Yes," Heather said weakly. "I begged him not to."

"I know it's difficult for you to think it, or even say the word, but when someone uses force—forces you to have sex with him against your will—that's rape."

Marilyn Levy, *Putting Heather Together Again* (New York: Ballantine, 1989), 107.

One part of me was snuggling into Nicky's warmth, but the skittery part of me inside was saying, No, this is your uncle, he's not a boyfriend, he's not your age, you shouldn't be wrapped here in his arms. But it was easy to pretend, as I stared into his eyes, that everything was all right. Nicky *was* a loving person. I hadn't seen him in so long. He was the closest male in my life now. . . .

      Michael Borich, *A Different Kind of Love*
      (New York: Holt, Rinehart and Winston,
               1985), 89.

Each of these passages represents a fictitious, but realistic, account of an incident involving unwanted sexual contact. In *Did You Hear What Happened to Andrea?*, Andrea is raped by a stranger who threatens her with a gun. Heather, in *Putting Heather Together Again*, is a victim of date rape. In *A Different Kind of Love*, Weeble becomes involved in an incestuous relationship with her uncle.

None of these teenage girls wants these sexual contacts, yet each of them suffers and feels she is to blame. Fortunately, each of these teenage victims tells someone about the situation. They all receive emotional support and professional counseling, which enable them to cope with the tragedy. Unfortunately, however, these fictitious cases of unwanted sexual contact reflect real-life tragedies for many contemporary teens.

- "It is estimated that one-third to almost one-half of all young people in the United States are sexually assaulted by the time they are eighteen. This could be by a stranger, acquaintance, date, or relative" (Grossman, 49).

Stranger rape, acquaintance rape, date rape, and incest are all forms of unwanted sexual contact. They involve some type of touching of the genitals, breasts, mouth, or other parts of the body associated with sexuality, against the will or without the consent of both people involved. Unwanted sexual contact can be broken down into two major categories: sexual assault and sexual abuse.

Sexual Assault

The term sexual assault covers a wide variety of forced sexual behaviors. Sexual assault is defined as any effort to force someone, against his or her will, into sexual intercourse or other sexual acts. A sexual assault is not an act of love; it is an aggressive act that involves sex.

WHO IS INVOLVED?

A study based on the results of the National Youth Survey (NYS) conducted between 1976 and 1980, using a nationally representative sample of teenagers, reveals the following information about teenagers and sexual assault:

- There are approximately 1 million teenage victims of sexual assault in the United States each year (Ageton, 4).
- Most sexual assault victims are females and most sexual assault offenders are male (ibid., 3).
- Teens from different racial backgrounds or social classes are equally involved with sexual assault, either as victims or offenders (ibid.).
- Adolescents who live in urban areas are more likely to be involved with sexual assault than those who live in suburban or rural areas (ibid.).
- The risk of involvement with sexual assault is greater among teens who have gotten into trouble for drinking and drug use and whose friends have done the same (ibid.).

In another study, the *Ms.* Foundation for Education and Communication surveyed 6,100 undergraduate males and females on 32 U.S. college campuses. This study provides information about the ages of women and men involved in rapes.

- "38 percent of the women who had been raped were 14, 15, 16, or 17 years old" (Warshaw, 117).
- "For both men and women, the average age when a rape occurred (either as a perpetrator or a victim) was 18½ years old" (ibid., 24).

TYPES OF SEXUAL ASSAULT

Although sexual assault can involve any objectionable touching of one person's body by another, rape is the most serious form of sexual assault.

- Rape is a highly significant problem that will affect approximately one in four women in their lifetimes (Parrot, 14).

Rape can be narrowly defined as forcing a male's penis into a female's vagina (vaginal intercourse), or it can be broadly defined as any forced sex act, including vaginal, oral, or anal penetration with a penis, hand, or other object. Many courts and counselors use the broad definition of the term, considering rape to be any sexual act in which one partner is unwilling and does not give consent. Using the broader definition means a sexual assault upon a male can be defined as rape, making both males and females potential rape victims. The broader definition is used in this chapter as the different types of rape are examined.

Forcible rape. Forcible rape is forced intercourse with a person of any age when the offender threatens or uses physical force, violence, or coercion. Use or threats of force may involve a weapon, or they may be verbal descriptions of what the offender will do if the victim does not comply. In either case, the victim has not consented to the sexual act and is an unwilling participant. In most states, having sexual intercourse out of fear for one's life or safety is legally defined as rape.

Statutory rape. Statutory rape is intercourse with someone who is below the age of consent, whether he or she agrees to have intercourse or not. The age of consent, which varies from state to state, usually falls between the ages of 16 and 18. Anyone having sex with someone under the age of consent can be charged with rape, even if both partners participate willingly. An exception is made to this law when the people involved are married to each other.

Stranger rape. Stranger rape is premeditated rape by someone who does not know the victim. This type of rape is most frequently reported to the police (ibid., 5), so it is the type we probably hear about most often. Police report that people who convey a sense of passivity or who seem easily intimidated are most attractive to stranger rapists (Bell, 130).

The appeal of rape to these offenders is not sexual gratification, but the sense of power they have over their victims. Physical violence and the use of weapons, therefore, are often part of the stranger rape situation. Statistics reporting the frequency of stranger rape involving adolescent victims are unavailable because information on adult rape and adolescent rape are generally not recorded separately.

Acquaintance rape. Acquaintance rape is forced sexual intercourse between two people who know each other.

- Although acquaintance rape can happen any time, it is most likely to occur during the teen years (ibid., 21).

The acquaintances involved may include neighbors, friends of the family, employers, coaches, ministers, teachers, or other adults or peers who have contact with the teen. Teenagers' inexperience in dealing with sexual situations makes them particularly susceptible to acquaintance rape. In addition, adolescent females with low self-esteem, who do not clearly communicate what is acceptable and unacceptable, and who engage in stereotypical female behaviors like flirting, indecisiveness, and manipulation, are more vulnerable for acquaintance rape than are more assertive young women (ibid., 16).

Date rape. Date rape, a type of acquaintance rape, is forced sexual intercourse that occurs between a dating couple or while on a date. It is the type of sexual assault most frequently reported in the NYS, so more information exists about this than about other rape circumstances. According to the NYS,

- "The typical teenage sexual assault is committed by a boyfriend or acquaintance and occurs during a date" (Ageton, iii).
- "Most assaults among teenagers do not involve severe physical violence or the use of a weapon" (ibid.).
- "The kind of force typically used is verbal pressure" (ibid.).
- "Often, drinking or drug use by the offender plays a part in causing the assault" (ibid.).

In most teenage date rape situations both the victim and the offender are adolescents. Because it is a type of acquaintance rape, the same dynamics operate to make certain types of females more vulnerable than others; girls who are unsure of themselves and think they should be submissive and try to please their dates are high risks for becoming acquaintance rape victims. Boys who believe the myth that all females want to be raped and that when they say no they really mean yes are likely to become offenders.

Unlike stranger rapes, most date rapes are not premeditated. A common pattern is that the male may expect to have sex during his date. He does not expect to rape his date, but when she does not consent, he forces her into it. The force may take the form of verbal pressure, like threatening to leave her alone in a secluded spot, or it may be more physically violent, like grasping her around the neck. Alcohol and drugs often accompany date rape; having intercourse with a female who is too drunk or high on drugs to understand what is happening to her is also considered rape, because the victim is unable to give her consent.

Homosexual rape. Males sometimes rape other males. The male victim may or may not be homosexual himself. Homosexual rapes, like heterosexual rapes, may be perpetrated by strangers or by acquaintances. They may also be forcible or statutory. Under the narrow definition of rape, forced homosexual contact is referred to as sexual assault or sodomy. Under the broader definition, this type of sexual assault is considered rape.

RAPE AND THE LAW

All rape is illegal. No one has the right to violate another person sexually. If both parties do not consent to the sexual act, it is rape. If one party says no, and the other forces sexual intercourse, it is rape.

No one deserves to be raped, no matter what he or she may say or do. The person who forces sex is responsible for the rape. Laws regarding rape, however, differ from state to state, so sometimes definitions of rape will influence the possibility of the offender's being convicted.

AFTER THE RAPE

A person who is raped has difficult decisions to make. He or she must decide whether to report the rape to the police and prosecute the offender. This decision is often clouded by confusion. Many victims feel they are somehow to blame for the rape, or they feel guilty or ashamed and don't want anyone to know what they have experienced. Often they do not want to admit they have experienced rape. Sometimes they need time to think and see the situation in a clearer perspective.

As with most traumatic occurrences, discussing the situation with a supportive relative, friend, religious counselor, or trained professional can ease the burden. Most communities have rape-crisis centers and rape hotlines that offer counseling and support to rape victims and those who care about them. It is never too late to take advantage of these support systems. The decision to use them can be made immediately or years later, although most professionals would suggest that the sooner the victim gets help, the better.

Rape victims must also decide if they want to utilize the legal system. Like decisions involving emotional support, this one does not have to be made right away, but the sooner it is, the fresher the evidence. When victims report rape, an officer, usually but not always a female, will advise them of their legal rights. If they decide to press charges, the officer will take the statement, collect evidence, and turn it over to the district attorney who will begin legal proceedings.

Part of the physical evidence the police will need comes from a medical examination of the victim. (See Chapter 3.) If possible, this exam should be administered within 72 hours after the rape in order to detect proof of forced intercourse. Female victims will also be tested for pregnancy and sexually transmitted diseases. Whether or not the victim decides to press charges, the medical examination ensures that no physical problems have gone unnoticed.

RAPE TRAUMA SYNDROME

Many rape victims experience the rape trauma syndrome as described by Andrea Parrot in *Coping with Date Rape & Acquaintance Rape*. The rape trauma syndrome has three phases: the acute or crisis phase, the disorientation phase, and the reorientation phase.

The crisis phase immediately follows the rape and may last days or even longer. At this time victims may be calm because they are in shock, or upset because they feel angry or guilty, or they may feel inappropriately carefree. Victims in the crisis stage often report feeling powerlessness, fear, anxiety, shame, embarrassment, shock, guilt, depression, and/or disbelief.

In the disorientation stage, victims are not sure how to act; they may have trouble interacting with other people. They may try to repress the memory of the rape and avoid getting in situations where it could happen again. Often they fear leaving their homes and limit their activities and the people with whom they interact.

In the reorientation phase, victims feel stronger and have gained a sense of how and why the rape happened. They begin to make constructive changes in their lives and regain some control and freedom. They are able to incorporate the memory of the rape into their lives and work for a positive future. Counseling and emotional support from others help most victims reach this final stage of healing, but some victims never reach it and remain in the disorientation phase, trying to repress the memory of their traumatic experience (Parrot, 43–44).

AVOIDING RAPE

While fear of stranger rape is certainly justified, it is important to keep in mind that most rapes involving teenagers occur between nonstrangers.

- Teenage girls are more likely to be sexually assaulted by a friend or date than a stranger (Ageton, 9).

Although it is never the victim's fault when rape occurs, rape may sometimes be prevented. NYS researcher Ageton offers the following suggestions to female teens:

- Check your own behavior for any unintentional sexual messages.
- Maintain control of your own behavior by not getting drunk or high on drugs.
- Be alert to sexual cues from your date or others.
- Clearly communicate your sexual limits.
- React immediately and negatively to unwanted sexual pressure.
- When selecting dates, be aware that teenage males who have delinquent backgrounds or friends are more likely to commit sexual assault than those who have not been in trouble with the law.
- Remember that most teenage males will not become violent or continue their attempts if you are firm in your refusal (ibid., 10–11).

Because they are frequently the offenders in teenage date rape cases, Ageton provides the following suggestions for teenage males:

- Don't assume that any flirtatious behavior is a signal for sex.

- Always respect the right of your date or partner to set her own sexual limits.
- Remember your date has a right to change her mind, just as you do.
- Discourage your friends from sexually aggressive behavior (ibid., 12).

Ageton reminds both males and females that they can do their part toward preventing sexual assault by remembering:

- *Everyone* has the right to say no to unwanted sexual contact.
- *No one* has the right to force sexual contact on another person (ibid.).

OTHER FORMS OF SEXUAL ASSAULT

Although rape is the most serious form of sexual assault, adolescents may also be victims of other forms of sexual attacks. Sexual assault may take the form of physical violence, like grabbing another's genitals or breast, or inflicting harm with a knife or other weapon. Sexual assault may also involve verbal force or threats, as when an offender demands that a teen undress or forces the victim to look at or touch the offender's genitals. Like rape, these types of sexual assault are illegal and the offender may be legally prosecuted.

Sexual Abuse

The second major category of unwanted sexual contact is sexual abuse. Unlike sexual assault, which usually involves some sort of violent attack to force sexual behavior, sexual abuse generally entails an older person pressuring a younger person into doing something sexual. The pressure is not so much violent as it is persuasive (Bell, 133).

Unlike victims of sexual assault, sexual abuse victims are not always unwilling. They may enjoy the attentions of the older, more powerful person or the tangible rewards given for sexual compliance and for keeping their secret. On the other hand, some victims participate unwillingly in order to hide their involvement, for which they feel guilty and somehow responsible, or to protect a loved one from harm initiated by the abuser. As in the case of sexual assault, teenagers can be both sexual abuse victims and offenders.

TYPES OF SEXUAL ABUSE

Incest. When sexual abuse, or molesting, occurs between people who are too closely related to be married to each other, it is called incest. Incest may include anything from touching, feeling, or kissing the sex organs to sexual intercourse. Children as well as teenagers can be involved with incest.

- "For every 100,000 adolescents in the general population, a minimum of 32.9 are victims of incest" (Burgess, 9).

Most victims of incest are girls. They are molested by their fathers, stepfathers, brothers, grandfathers, uncles, or older brothers. Boys are less frequently molested by male relatives. Incest between mothers and sons or mothers and daughters occurs the least frequently of all.

Brothers and sisters often engage in sex play when they are children. Most people agree that playing doctor, for example, is a harmless activity as long as one child does not coerce another into doing something that makes him or her feel uncomfortable.

The problem comes when older siblings use the power associated with their size or age to pressure a younger sibling into an incestuous relationship.

Adults too use their size and natural authority over children and teenagers to make them submit to incest. Incest victims frequently feel confused about their situation. They commonly believe they did something to cause the adult's behavior and also think they will be punished if others learn what is occurring. They may also be intimidated by the abuser or they may wish to protect him because he is a family member. For reasons like these, the victim often keeps the behavior of the relative a dark family secret.

Child Molesting. A relative who touches, feels, kisses, or penetrates a child or teenager's sexual organs is guilty of incest. A nonfamily member who engages in these behaviors is guilty of child molesting.

Child molesters are usually not strangers, but people whom children or teenagers know and trust, like close family friends, babysitters, school-bus drivers, physicians, leaders of boys' and girls' activity groups, and neighbors (Ledray, 148). Child molesters who are not strangers use the same types of pressure to persuade the victim to comply and keep their secret. They may offer rewards or issue threats, but they rely upon their power as an elder to make the victim obey.

DISCLOSING CHILD ABUSE

- "Incest or child molesting by a trusted friend is often more devastating than molestation by a stranger" (ibid., 149).

It is often more difficult for victims of incest or child molesting by nonstrangers to disclose what has happened than it is for victims of strangers. Victims do not feel any loyalty toward strangers and may not feel the guilt and shame as intensely as they may with nonstrangers. In any case, however, it is only when the victim reveals the secret of incest or child abuse that there is any chance to rectify the situation.

Victims may find the strength to confide in a trusted friend or relative, or they may choose to talk to a professional counselor. Contacting a child-abuse hotline may be a first step for a victim. People who do not disclose that they have been molested carry the secret with them long after the abusive relationship has ended.

EFFECTS OF SEXUAL ABUSE

The effects of sexual abuse are both immediate and long-term. During the time a child or teenager is being sexually abused, he or she may have difficulty relating to other people. Victims may fear discovery of their situation or distrust intimate relationships and therefore limit their interactions with peers and adults. They may not be able to engage in healthy relationships with the opposite sex.

Without some kind of professional counseling or therapy, victims will most likely experience problems related to the abuse throughout their lifetimes. They may always have difficulty in relationships with the opposite sex and frequently select partners who are abusive. They may also become abusive themselves.

- Children or teenagers who were themselves victims of sexual abuse very often become child abusers (ibid., 148).

Help for Victims of Unwanted Sexual Contact

Unwanted sexual contact, whether it be sexual assault or sexual abuse, is a traumatic experience. However, as professionals learn more about the people involved, either as victims or offenders, they gain insight into how to help these people. Many of the effects can be overcome, and the victims who have survived these situations often become mentally healthy members of society.

But help only comes after the problem has been identified. Reporting unwanted sexual contact is the first step toward overcoming the effects of rape, sexual assault, incest, or child molesting.

REFERENCES

Ageton, Suzanne S. *A Research Report for Teenagers*. Rockville, MD: U.S. Department of Health and Human Services, 1985.

Bell, Ruth, et al. *Changing Bodies, Changing Lives: A Book for Teens on Sex and Relationships.* New York: Random House, 1987.

Burgess, Ann Wolvert. *The Sexual Victimization of Adolescents.* Washington, DC: U.S. Government Printing Office, 1985.

Grossman, Rochel, with Joan Sutherland. *Surviving Sexual Assault.* New York: Congdon & Weed, 1983.

Ledray, Linda E. *Recovering from Rape.* New York: Henry Holt, 1986.

Parrot, Andrea. *Coping with Date Rape & Acquaintance Rape.* New York: Rosen Publishing Group, 1988.

Warshaw, Robin. *I Never Called It Rape: The Ms. Report on Recognizing, Fighting and Surviving Date and Acquaintance Rape.* New York: Harper & Row, 1988.

Resources
for Finding Out about Unwanted Sexual Contact

Unwanted Sexual Contact in Fiction

These young-adult novels present various perspectives on rape, incest, and child molesting. Some offer recent treatments of these topics in young-adult literature, while others have a more historical view.

Borich, Michael. **A Different Kind of Love.** New York: Holt, Rinehart and Winston (New American Library), 1985. 165p.

Fourteen-year-old Elizabeth (Weeble) is popular, a cheerleader, and gets along well with her mother and her teachers. But there is something missing in her life. She never knew her father and has no one to play that special role. Then her uncle Nicky, whom she has not seen for eight years, comes to visit.

Nicky is 25, a rock star, kind, attractive, and quite attentive to Weeble. Weeble turns to him for the love and support she would like from a father. But the love Nicky has for Weeble is the romantic sort, and Weeble feels confused and guilty. She asks her friends for advice and finally tells her mother about the situation. Her mother confronts Nicky and he leaves.

Crutcher, Chris. **Chinese Handcuffs.** New York: Morrow, 1989. 202p.

High school junior Jennifer Lawless is pretty, a 4.0 student, and a basketball star. As a young child, she was sexually abused by her father. After seeing the film *Good Touch, Bad*

Touch, Jennifer tells on her father and he leaves. Jennifer's mother remarries, but her stepfather rapes her. He continues to sexually abuse her, threatening to kill her puppy or harm her sister and mother if she reveals the secret. When Jennifer can stand it no longer, she tells her friend Dillon Hemingway, who is evenutally able to help her.

Along with a compelling story, this novel provides detailed information about the psychology of incest.

Dizenzo, Patricia. **Why Me? The Story of Jenny.** New York: Avon, 1976. 142p.

Jenny, 15, is raped by a stranger from whom she accepts a ride on a cold night. She does not tell her parents for fear that they will not believe her. She only tells one friend, who does not seem to be of any help. All alone, she copes with a visit to a clinic and the system of venereal disease tests. She waits nervously for her period.

Finally, she tells her mother about the incident. When her mother tells Jenny's father, he explodes and shows his anger by lashing out at Jenny. Later he tells Jenny he is not angry with her, but at the situation she put herself in and at the man who raped his little girl. Following the advice of her parents and a school counselor, Jenny gets help to deal with her trauma. Jenny's story talks about the lonely feeling that a rape victim can suffer and the fear of telling others. Jenny was afraid that she would not be believed and that she would be blamed.

Hermes, Patricia. **A Solitary Secret.** New York: Harcourt Brace Jovanovich, 1985. 135p.

The 14-year-old protagonist, or central character, in this story remains unnamed. Her mother deserts her, leaving the girl with her cruel father. The father sexually abuses his daughter, causing her to question why this is happening, what she should do, whether she is pregnant, and how to get out of the terrible situation. After the death of her only real friend, Sheila, the protagonist reveals her secret to Sheila's mother and no longer has to bear her burden alone.

Irwin, Hadley. **Abby, My Love.** New York: Atheneum, 1985. 157p.

This is a compelling story about a seventh-grade girl, Abby, who is keeping a very serious secret. Her father has been sexually abusing her since she was a young child. She used to believe it was all a bad dream. Now, she is older and she knows the truth.

Chip is infatuated with Abby, but she confuses him. Sometimes she is friendly and sometimes she is withdrawn. Abby is terrified when she learns that her mother and sister are going out of town for a weekend and leaving her alone with her father. Finally, she confides in Chip and eventually goes to a child protection agency and files a complaint against her father. This story realistically explores many facets of the effects of incest.

Levy, Marilyn. **Putting Heather Together Again.** New York: Ballantine (Fawcett Juniper), 1989. 136p.

Seventeen-year-old Heather is beautiful, but lacks self-confidence. When her boyfriend, Vince, breaks up with her, she reluctantly begins to date Joe, who is three years older than she. Heather becomes a victim of date rape when Joe takes her to his friend's house, gets her drunk, ignores her protests, and has sex with her. Heather feels terrible about losing her virginity, but believes it was her fault for being "stupid."

She finally tells her stepmother what happened. Her stepmother takes Heather to a rape crisis center to talk to a counselor. Heather undergoes a gynecological exam, which the author describes, and is tested for STDs. Heather's stepmother admits that she had a similar experience when she was young. Heather continues to see the therapist, and with the love and support of her family, eventually tells Vince what happened to her.

Miklowitz, Gloria D. **Did You Hear What Happened to Andrea?** New York: Delacorte (Dell), 1978. 168p.

Fifteen-year-old Andrea Cranston is raped by a man who picks her up hitchhiking. In this novel, Miklowitz confronts the topic of stranger rape from a new angle. She reveals the feelings of each of the people involved: the victim, her parents, her friends, her boyfriend. The story effectively deals with the issue of self-blame and how rape victims can overcome this feeling. Andrea stuggles to regain her self-image and finds that the only way she will be able to face herself is by bringing her attacker to court and getting him convicted. The book makes strong recommendations about effective ways of dealing with the tragedy of rape.

Miklowitz, Gloria D. **Secrets Not Meant To Be Kept.** New York: Delacorte (Dell), 1987. 138p.

Adri worries because she seems to respond abnormally to the affections of her boyfriend, Ryan. Instead of being pleased by his physical attentions, she stiffens up, feels nauseous, and loses her breath. She also worries about her three-year-old sister, who experiences terrible nightmares. Adri suspects her sister is being molested at her nursery school, the same one Adri attended, although she remembers nothing of her life before she was six or seven. Adri discovers that she too was molested at the nursery school. Adri understands her own problems better and realizes she must do something to stop the sexual abuse that continues at the preschool.

Peck, Richard. **Are You in the House Alone?** New York: Viking (Dell), 1976. 172p.

This novel focuses on a specific kind of rape, acquaintance rape. Gail is raped by her best friend's boyfriend. She is tormented for weeks by unsigned, explicitly disgusting notes and frightening telephone calls. After the rape, Gail spends days in the hospital and weeks at home in bed. She would like to bring her attacker up on charges, but she believes this process would be pointless because the rapist is the son of the wealthiest, most prominent man in Oldfield Village.

The book effectively describes the phases that a rape victim goes through in dealing with her situation. Acquaintance rape is a new term for an old problem, and the author does a nice job of describing the victim's feelings toward her attacker and how she deals with seeing him daily in school.

Scoppettone, Sandra. **Happy Endings Are All Alike.** New York: Harper & Row (Dell), 1978. 202p.

Jaret and Peggy, recent high school graduates, have been lovers for several months. One of the few people who knows they are lesbians is Mid Summers, a disturbed teenage boy who hates Jaret because she pays no attention to him. Mid bides his time and spies on the couple. One day when Jaret is alone in the woods, Mid assaults and rapes her. He threatens to reveal her homosexuality if she reports him. Jaret's family finds her in the woods and takes her to the hospital. Jaret reports Mid and decides to press charges.

Nonfiction Materials on Unwanted Sexual Contact

The following sources represent the types of information available on unwanted sexual contact. Many of these sources were written specifically for teenage readers. Others contain sections for or about adolescents. Those that may be too scholarly for teens are noted.

BOOKS AND PAMPHLETS

Adams, Caren, and Jennifer Fay. **"Nobody Told Me It Was Rape": A Parent's Guide for Talking with Teenagers about Acquaintance Rape and Sexual Exploitation.** Santa Cruz, CA: Network Publications, 1984. 25p.

This is a handbook to help parents communicate with their teenagers about the topics of rape, acquaintance rape, and sexual exploitation. The guide discusses how one could become a victim or a victimizer, the force involved in rape, the effects of rape on a teenager, prevention ideas, and how to set limits. This booklet is easy to read and provides useful information for teens as well as their parents.

Ageton, Suzanne S. **A Research Report for Teenagers: Facts about Sexual Assault.** Rockville, MD: U.S. Department of

Health and Human Services, National Institute of Mental Health, 1985. 15p.

This report on sexual assault, written for adolescents, contains data on teenage sexual assault from the National Youth Survey (NYS). About 1,700 youths between 11 and 17 years old were interviewed annually for five years (1976 to 1980) for the survey. The data about sexual assault were obtained from self-identified victims and offenders. The research study is briefly described and findings from it are used to answer some common questions teenagers ask about sexual assault.

The report is straightforward and easy to read. Much of its emphasis is on date rape. Advice is given to both boys and girls on how to prevent a sexual assault. The author, a member of the research team, wrote the report under a grant from the National Center for the Prevention and Control of Rape, National Institute of Mental Health.

Bell, Ruth, et al. **Changing Bodies, Changing Lives: A Book for Teens on Sex and Relationships.** New York: Random House (Vintage), 1987. 254p.

A section on sex against your will is included in this comprehensive book on teen sexuality and general health. It was written specifically for teenagers with teens' views on their own sexuality included. The authors write in a frank manner and provide a range of perspectives on the topic. This is one of the best resources available for teens.

Eagan, Andrea Boroff. **Why Am I So Miserable If These Are the Best Years of My Life?: Everything Your Mother Never Told You about Becoming a Woman.** New York: Avon, 1988. 211p.

Among the wide variety of topics of concern to adolescents is legal rights. Information about rape and incest is included in one section. Eagan presents the facts and gives advice in this easily readable guide for young women.

Fay, Jennifer J., and Billie Jo Flerchinger. **Top Secret: Sexual Assault Information for Teenagers Only.** Renton, WA: King County Rape Relief, 1983. 85p.

Written exclusively for teenagers, this booklet about rape is easy, interesting, and informative. First-person stories about rape, and question and answer sections modeled after the "Dear Abby" format are included. Advice is given in an interesting, subtle way. The information is valuable, precise, and even enjoyable to read.

Grossman, Rochel, ed., with Joan Sutherland. **Surviving Sexual Assault.** New York: Congdon & Weed, 1983. 85p.

This booklet was prepared at the request of hospital emergency-room personnel by the Los Angeles Commission on Assaults against Women and the National Council of Jewish Women, Los Angeles. In a very readable format, it answers questions asked by women who have been assaulted. It also gives tips on the prevention of assault, information for the friends and family of assault survivors, and a nationwide directory of rape-crisis centers and hotlines. A special section is addressed to teens who have been sexually assaulted.

Hughes, Jean Ogorman, and Bernice R. Sandler. **"Friends" Raping Friends: Could It Happen to You?** Washington, DC: Project on the Status and Education of Women, Association of American Colleges, 1987. 8p.

Although this booklet is written with college students in mind, it contains excellent information and advice for high school students as well. Date rape is defined and its usual patterns and causes are explained. Suggestions on ways to avoid date rape and what to do if it happens are provided, along with a list of the effects and legal implications of date rape.

Johnson, Eric W. **Love & Sex in Plain Language.** Philadelphia: Lippincott (Bantam), 1985. 207p.

Originally written in 1968, this comprehensive but concise book is in its fourth revision. Along with other topics related to sex and sexuality, the author discusses ways sex can be a problem. This book is not difficult to read. Illustrations, glossary, and an index make the contents accessible.

Ledray, Linda E. **Recovering from Rape.** New York: Henry Holt, 1986. 258p.

Although not written specifically for or about teens, this book could be a useful resource. The author, a registered nurse who has a Ph.D., covers the topics of rape and childhood sexual abuse thoroughly, knowledgeably, and compassionately. She writes for both the survivor of rape and the survivor's significant others. A comprehensive list of rape-crisis centers across the United States is included along with a list of suggested readings. Half of the author's earnings from *Recovering from Rape* are donated to the Sexual Assault Resource Service and to the National Coalition against Sexual Assault.

Madaras, Lynda, with Area Madaras. **The What's Happening to My Body? Book for Girls: A Growing Up Guide for Parents and Daughters.** New York: Newmarket, 1988. 269p.

Written especially for younger adolescents and their parents, this book primarily focuses on female puberty, but the authors include brief sections on rape, incest, and child molesting. The frank, clear explanations and conversational writing style make information on sexual development accessible to the intended audience. Illustrations enhance the text, and an index is included.

Madaras, Lynda, with Dane Saavedra. **The What's Happening to My Body? Book for Boys: A Growing Up Guide for Parents and Sons.** New York: Newmarket, 1987. 251p.

Written by a sex educator with the assistance of a teenage boy, the primary topic of this book is male puberty. The authors include brief sections on rape, incest, and child molesting. The tone is honest and conversational. The intended audience is younger adolescents and their parents. An index and illustrations are included.

Parrot, Andrea. **Coping with Date Rape & Acquaintance Rape.** New York: Rosen Publishing Group, 1988. 134p.

Written for male and female adolescents by one of the country's leading sex educators, this book discusses the issue of date and acquaintance rape in a straightforward, informative manner. The book speaks to females and males who have been victims of date or acquaintance rape, helping them understand their feelings and rights. It also discusses ways males and females can prevent date and acquaintance rape. The book includes case studies taken from interviews of rape victims, a glossary, bibliography, index, and list of human resources. This is an excellent resource, providing information not only about rape, but also about sexual decision making and physical aspects of sexuality.

Ward, Elizabeth. **Father-Daughter Rape.** New York: Grove Press, 1985. 247p.

This book spotlights the crime of incest. Part one consists of nine factual and sometimes disturbing accounts, including incest committed by father, brother, grandfather, and mother's boyfriend. Part two discusses the Freudian theory behind incest. Part three details actions that must be taken against incest. This scholarly treatment of the subject would be appropriate for adults interested in a thorough, theoretical approach to the topic.

Warshaw, Robin. **I Never Called It Rape: The *Ms.* Report on Recognizing, Fighting and Surviving Date and Acquaintance Rape.** New York: Harper & Row, 1988. 229p.

Using a college-based survey on acquaintance rape sponsored by the *Ms.* Foundation for Education and Communication, along with scholarly information and personal accounts from rape survivors, Warshaw explains what date rape is, how it happens, why it goes unreported, how the legal system responds, and how it can be prevented. She also describes the men who commit acquaintance rape and the benefits of change for men. There is a special chapter on teenagers and acquaintance rape. A list of resources, including videotapes, an index, and an extensive bibliography are included.

Weston, Carol. **Girltalk about Guys.** New York: Harper & Row, 1988. 220p.

Structuring her information around real letters from teens, Weston devotes two-thirds of this book to relationship topics. In a brief section, she discusses unwanted sexual contact. The information given is solid, and the advice shows a genuine caring for teens. The author's chatty style makes the information easy to read and her advice easy to consider.

Wong, Debbie, and Scott Wittet. **Be Aware. Be Safe.** Renton, WA: Washington State Department of Social and Health Services, 1987. 38p.

This illustrated booklet on sexual assault was designed especially for Southeast Asian teenagers. Three stories illustrate sexual assault cases. Topics covered include dating, the definition of sexual assault, offenders, the effects and prevention of sexual assault, and what to do after a sexual assault. The text is in English, with a short glossary that translates key words into Vietnamese, Chinese, Cambodian, and Lao. Several quizzes are provided.

Nonprint Materials on Unwanted Sexual Contact

The following films and videos address the topic of unwanted sexual contact. These materials are geared toward teenage audiences. Reviewing sources included *Lander's Film Review, Video Source Book, Media Review Digest,* and *School Library Booklist.*

Acquaintance Rape Series
Type: 4 VHS videocassettes
Length: 30 min. each
Cost: Purchase $180 each
Distributor: Great Plains National Instructional TV Library
Box 80669
Lincoln, NE 68501
Date: 1980

The aim of this film series is to prevent rape among people who know each other.

Child Lures I: Training and Prevention of Molestation and Abduction
Type: Videocassette
Length: 45 min.
Cost: Purchase $150–190
Distributor: Landmark Films
               3450 Slade Run Drive
               Falls Church, VA 22042
Date: 1986

Common lures that possible abductors and molestors use to abduct children are discussed. The video concentrates on instructing children from various age groups.

Child Sexual Abuse: What Your Children Should Know Series: A Program for Senior High
Type: 16mm film, VHS videocassette
Length: 60 min.
Cost: Rental $35; purchase $635 (film), $250 (video)
Distributor: Indiana University Audio-Visual Center
               Bloomington, IN 47405
Date: 1983

The last in a four-part series, this film deals with understanding factors involved in sexual assault and minimizing the risk. In a discussion lead by Billie Jo Flerchinger of King County Rape Relief, high school students talk about how sexual assault happens, who the victims are, and who the assailants are. They learn to anticipate the kinds of situations that can lead to sexual assault and discuss how to minimize those risks.

Child Sexual Abuse Prevention: Socio-cultural and Community Issues
Type: VHS or Beta videocassette
Length: 30 min.
Cost: Rental $50; purchase $145

Distributor: AIMS Media
6901 Woodley Avenue
Van Nuys, CA 91406-4878
Date: 1986

This video is part of an educational package for teachers and parents that is designed to teach children of any age about preventing sexual abuse.

Date Rape
Type: VHS videocassette
Length: 48 min.
Cost: Purchase $225
Distributor: Intermedia
1300 Dexter Avenue North
Seattle, WA 98109
Date: 1988

Told from a male perspective, this video looks at beliefs, deeply rooted in our society, that encourage young men to oversubscribe to traditional male attitudes that say aggression is normal and males have to prove themselves by demonstrating their virility. As the teenage narrator tells how he committed date rape, viewers come to understand the damaging effects the act has on both males and females.

Presenting a Personal Safety Curriculum
Type: VHS videocassette
Length: 30 min.
Cost: Rental $50; purchase $145
Distributor: AIMS Media
6901 Woodley Avenue
Van Nuys, CA 91406-4878
Date: 1986

This video demonstrates lessons in personal safety.

Sexual Abuse and Harassment: Causes, Prevention . . . Coping
Type: VHS videocassette
Length: 60 min.
Cost: Purchase $209

Distributor: Guidance Associates, Inc.
Communications Park, P.O. Box 3000
Mt. Kisco, NY 10549
Date: 1986

Different types of sexual abuse are explored and methods are suggested for avoiding and overcoming them. Counselors and former victims are interviewed.

Someone You Know
Type: VHS videocassette
Length: 29 min.
Cost: Rental $35; purchase $295
Distributor: Perennial Education, Inc.
930 Pitner Avenue
Evanston, IL 60202
Date: 1989

This program about date and acquaintance rape is designed to stimulate discussion through two very realistic situations. One involves a victim of date rape; the other involves a victim of gang rape at a college house party. A man and a woman discuss their reactions to each situation.

Someone You Know: Acquaintance Rape
Type: 16mm film, VHS videocassette
Length: 30 min.
Cost: Rental $125; purchase $550 (film), $470 (video)
Distributor: Coronet/MTI Films
108 Wilmot Road
Deerfield, IL 60015-9990
Date: 1986

Hosted by Collin Siedor, the film explores the magnitude of the date rape problem. Sound bites from a call to police during an actual rape, interviews with women who have been raped, and interviews with sex offenders are presented.

Stop Date Rape
Type: VHS videocassette
Length: 20 min.
Cost: Rental $50; purchase $225

Distributor: Cornell University Media Services
Audio Visual Resource Center
8 Research Park
Ithaca, NY 14850
Date: 1987

Two scenarios are shown: one ends in date rape; date rape is prevented in the other. Discussion is invited regarding the reasons for date rape.

Without Consent
Type: 16mm film, VHS videocassette
Length: 25 min.
Cost: Rental $65; purchase $475 (film), $295 (video)
Distributor: Pyramid Film and Video
Box 1048
Santa Monica, CA 90406
Date: 1987

This movie dramatizes a date rape involving two law students, and the ensuing discussions in their law school surrounding the issue of date rape.

Organizations Concerned with Unwanted Sexual Contact

If you have a crisis involving sexual assault, local organizations that can help you may be found in the telephone directory under one of these headings: Crisis Intervention Services, Human Service Organizations, Police or Sheriff Departments, Rape Crisis Centers, Sexual Assault Assistance Centers, Social Service Organizations, and Victim Assistance Organizations.

National Coalition against Sexual Assault (NCASA)
2428 Ontario Road NE
Washington, DC 20009
(202) 483-7165
Director: Claire Kaplan

NCASA is an umbrella organization that provides educational training, technical assistance, and support for rape-crisis centers throughout the nation. The telephone number listed above is an information/referral line. You may call it if you need information regarding local organizations concerned about rape, sexual assault, child abuse, or incest. You may also write to NCASA and request such information. While this is not a rape hotline, the operators could direct you to one in your area.

Hotline

Child Abuse Hotline   (800) 4A-CHILD

You may call this hotline at no charge to talk about any form of child abuse, including incest. The operators are trained to provide crisis counseling and referrals.

Index

Abby, My Love, 199
Abduction, videocassette on, 207
Abortion, 95–99
   in fiction, 110, 112, 114–117
   in nonfiction, 122
   videocassettes on, 127–129
Abstinence, 61–64, 87
Abuse, sexual, 192–195
   hotline for, 211
   nonfiction on, 204
   organization for, 210–211
   videocassettes on, 207–209
Acquaintance rape, 187–188
   in fiction, 81, 200–201
   nonfiction on, 23, 52, 201, 204–205
   videocassettes on, 206, 209
Acquaintance Rape Series, 206–207
Adams, Caren, 201
Adams, Gina, 106
Adler, C. S., 12, 79
Adoption, 102–104
   in fiction, 111–116
   hotline for, 134
   videocassette on, 127
Adoption Hotline, 134
Affinity, 33
Affirmation/Gay and Lesbian Mormons, 33
Agency adoptions, 103
Ageton, Suzanne S., 185, 188, 191–192, 201
AIDS, 68, 136–137, 144–147
   in fiction, 159–160
   hotlines for, 178–181
   nonfiction about, 160–166
   organizations for, 177–178
   videocassettes on, 167–171, 173–177
AIDS, 161, 167
AIDS: Answers for Young People, 167
AIDS: Changing the Rules, 167–168
AIDS: Facts and Fears, Crisis and Controversy, 168
AIDS: Facts over Fear, 168
AIDS: One Family's Story, 168
AIDS: The Facts, 163
AIDS: What Does It Mean to You?, 161
AIDS Alert for Youth, 169
AIDS Epidemic: Is Anyone Safe?, 169
AIDS Hits Home, 169
AIDS Hotline for Teens, 178
AIDS in Your School, 170
Alan Guttmacher Institute, 118
Alcohol and date rape, 188
Alyson, Sasha, 160
American Social Health Association, 177
Anal sex, 6
Anatomy Attitudes: Understanding Sexuality, 52–53
And Baby Makes Two: A Look at Teenage Single Parents, 123–124

Angel Face, 16–17
Annie on My Mind, 15
Another Half, 124
ARC (AIDS-related complex), 136–137, 145
Are You in the House Alone?, 200
Are You There God? It's Me, Margaret, 37–38, 49
The Arizona Kid, 17, 80, 159
Articles
  on contraception, 84
  on pregnancy, 123
  on sexually transmitted diseases, 166
Asner, Ed, 129
Assault, sexual, 185–192
  nonfiction on, 201–206
  See also Rape

Babies
  prenatal care for, 99–101
  sexuality of, 2
Bacteria, 149–154
Barr, Linda, 118
Be Aware. Be Safe, 206
Be Still My Heart, 158–159
Belief systems and contraceptives, 60
Bell, Ruth, 20–21, 50, 60, 82, 118, 120, 160, 192, 202
Berman, Claire, 123
Best Defense, 170
Bet Mispocheh, 33
Bet Mispocheh Newsletter, 33
Betancourt, Jeanne, 13, 79, 110
Beth Chayim Chadashim, 34
Binding Ties, 12, 79
Bird at the Window, 117
Birth
  and adoption, 102–104
  health concerns in, 99–101
Birth control. See Contraception
Birth Control Movie, 84
Bisexuality, 8
Blood tests
  for pregnancy, 94
  for sexually transmitted diseases, 139, 145–147, 153

Blood transfusions and AIDS, 136, 146
Blume, Judy, 13, 37, 49, 79, 110, 135, 158
Bode, Janet, 118
Bograd, Larry, 14, 58, 80
Bondings, 35
Bonnie Jo, Go Home, 112
Books. See Fiction; Nonfiction
Borich, Michael, 184, 197
Bowe-Gutman, Sonia, 119
Brandt, Pam, 123
Breast development, 45–46
Breast examinations, videocassette on, 86–87
Brethren/Mennonite Council for Lesbian and Gay Concerns, 34
Bridgers, Sue Ellen, 14, 57, 80
Bryson, Yvonne, 172
Burgess, Ann Wolvert, 193–195
Burt, Martha R., 121

Calendar birth-control method, 62–63
Calvert, Patricia, 111
"Can You Rely on Condoms?," 84, 166
Catholic Church
  and contraceptives, 60
  support for homosexuals within, 34–35
Centers for Disease Control, 177
Changing Bodies, Changing Lives: A Book for Teens on Sex and Relationships, 20–21, 50, 82, 118, 120, 160, 202
Child abuse, hotline for, 211
Child Lures I: Training and Prevention of Molestation and Abduction, 207
Child molesting, 194
  in fiction, 200
  videocassettes on, 207–208
Child Sexual Abuse: What Your Children Should Know Series: A Program for Senior High, 207

Child Sexual Abuse Prevention:
  Socio-cultural and
  Community Issues, 207–208
Child Welfare League of America, 132–133
Children, sexuality of, 2
Children of Children, 124
Chinese Handcuffs, 111, 197–198
Chlamydia, 151–152
Choices
  in pregnancy, 95–105
  in sexuality, 8–10
Choices, 170–171
Chong, Rae Dawn, 166, 174
Choosing To Wait: Sex and Teenagers, 24
Circumcision, 38–39
Clap, 149–151
Clitoris, 40
Close Encounters of the Sexual Kind, 171
Common Sexual Problems, 24
Communication, about STDs, 141
Complete abstinence, 61–62
Conception, 41–42
  prevention of. See Contraception
Condom Sense, 84–85
Condom-eze, 85
Condoms, 59, 65–66
  and sexually transmitted diseases, 68, 143, 146, 148, 150–151
  videocassette about, 171
Cone, Molly, 111
Consumer Reports, 84, 166
Contraception, 57
  abstinence, 61–64
  decisions about using, 58–61
  fallacies about, 77
  in fiction, 79–81
  nonfiction on, 81–84
  nonprescription methods of, 64–70
  nonprint materials on, 84–88
  organizations for, 88–89
  prescription methods for, 70–77
  and sexually transmitted diseases, 141
  videocassettes on, 31, 84–88

Contraceptive Choices, 85
Contraceptive Update, 85
Coping with Adolescence: Understanding Puberty, 53
Coping with AIDS: Facts and Fears, 162–163
Coping with Date Rape & Acquaintance Rape, 23, 52, 190–191, 204–205
Coping with Herpes Series: A Family of Viruses, 171
Coping with Herpes Series: Herpes and Long-Term Relationships, 171–172
Coping with Herpes Series: Herpes and Pregnancy, 172
Coping with Herpes Series: Herpes and Single People, 172
Coping with Herpes Series: Treatment and Management of Symptoms, 172
Counseling, rape, 189–191
Crab lice, 155
Cream contraceptives, 68–69, 144
Crisis: Heterosexual Behavior in the Age of AIDS, 164
Crutcher, Chris, 111, 197
Culture tests for STDs, 139

D & C abortions, 97–98
D & E abortions, 98
Date rape, 184, 187–188
  in fiction, 81, 199
  nonfiction on, 23, 52, 202–203
  videocassettes on, 208–210
Date Rape, 208
Dating: Coping with the Pressures, 24–25
Davis, Jenny, 1, 14, 50
Deciso 3003, 25
Deep kissing, 5
Delayed abortions, 98–99
Dementia, 145
Development. See Physical development
Dialogue, 34
Diaphragms, 73–74, 150

Did You Hear What Happened to Andrea, 183–184, 199–201
Diet during pregnancy, 101
Different Kind of Love, 184, 197
Dilation and curettage abortions, 97–98
Dilation and evacuation abortions, 98
Dizenzo, Patricia, 111, 158, 198
Don't Forget Sherri, 173
Don't Look and It Won't Hurt, 115
Drip (gonorrhea), 149–151
Dropping out of school from pregnancy, 106
Drug use
  AIDS from, 146, 165–166, 174
  and date rape, 188

Eagan, Andrea Boroff, 21, 50, 82, 119, 138, 161, 202
Egg, 41–42
Ejaculations, 3, 39–42, 44
Elfman, Blossom, 111–112
ELISA, 146–147
Emotions
  and pregnancy, 94–95
  after rape, 190–191
  and sexual development, 46–47
Enzyme-linked immunosorbent assay test, 146–147
An Epidemic of Teen Pregnancy? Some Historical and Policy Considerations, 122
Erections, 3, 39, 42, 49
Ewy, Donna, 119
Ewy, Rodger, 119
Examinations, physical, 70–73
  in fiction, 80–81
  after rape, 190
  for sexually transmitted diseases, 140
  videocassette on, 86–87
External genitals, 38–40
Eyerly, Jeannette, 112

Fallacies about birth control, 77
Fallopian tubes, 41–42
Family adoptions, 102
Father-Daughter Rape, 205
Fathers
  and pregnancy, 107–108
  videocassette on, 130
Fay, Jennifer J., 201–202
Fears and contraceptives, 60
Federation of Feminist Women's Health Centers, 133
Females
  reproductive system of, 40–41
  sexual development of, 42, 45–46
  sexual response of, 3–4
Fetal development, videocassette on, 54
Fiction
  contraception in, 79–81
  physical development in, 49–50
  pregnancy in, 110–117
  sexuality in, 12–20
  sexually transmitted diseases in, 158–160
  unwanted sexual contact in, 197–201
Fighting Back: What Some People Are Doing about AIDS, 162
Films and videocassettes
  on contraception, 84–88
  on physical development, 52–54
  on pregnancy, 123–132
  on sexuality, 23–32
  on sexually transmitted diseases, 167–177
  on unwanted sexual contact, 206–210
First Things First, 25
Flerchinger, Billie Jo, 202, 207
Foam contraceptive, 66–68
  and sexually transmitted diseases, 67–68, 144, 148, 150–151
Follicle-stimulating hormones, 45
For All the Wrong Reasons, 115
Forcible rape, 186
Forever, 13, 79–80, 110–111, 135–136, 158

Forrest, Jacqueline, 63
Forsyth, Elizabeth H., 161
Four Pregnant Teenagers: Four Different Decisions, 124–125
French-kissing, 5
"Friends" Raping Friends: Could It Happen to You?, 203

Garden, Nancy, 15
Gates, Joanne, 120
Gay Men's Health Crisis, 162
Gays. *See* Homosexuality
Genital herpes, 142–144
Genitals, 38–41
Getting Free, 113
A Girl Like Me, 112
The Girl of His Dreams, 18
Girl Stuff, 53
The Girls of Huntington House, 111–112
Girltalk about Guys, 23, 83, 122, 166, 206
Gladney Center, 133
Gonorrhea, 135, 149–151
Good-bye Tomorrow, 136, 159–160
Gramick, Jeannine, 34
Gram's stain test, 140
The Great Chastity Experiment, 25
Griffiths, Leslie, 161
Grimes, Tammy, 129
Grossman, Rochel, 184, 203
Growing Up in a Hurry, 114
Gulas, Ivan, 161
Gumbel, Bryant, 30
Guy, Rosa, 15
Gvanim, 34
Gynecological examinations, 70–73
   in fiction, 80–81
   for sexually transmitted diseases, 140
   videocassette on, 86–87

Hall, Lynn, 15
Hansen, Caryl, 113

Happy Endings Are All Alike, 19, 201
Hard Climb, 26
Hautzig, Deborah, 1, 16
Hawkes, Nigel, 161
Hayes, Cheryl D., 106, 120
Head, Ann, 113
Health
   and birth, 99–101
   and contraceptives, 59
   See also Sexually transmitted diseases
Hein, Karen, 4, 7–8, 60, 67, 73–76
Helper, 178
Henshaw, S. K., 92
Hepatitis B, 147–148
Hermes, Patricia, 158, 198
Heron, Ann, 7, 21
Herpes, 142–144
   hotline for, 178
   nonfiction on, 161, 165
   organization for, 177–178
   videocassettes on, 171–173
Herpes, 165
Herpes: The Love Bug: Facts and Fears, 161
Herpes Hotline, 178
Herpes Research Center, 177–178
"Herpie": The New VD around Town, 173
He's No Hero, 26
Heterosexuality, 7
Hey, Dollface, 1–2, 16
Hinton, Nigel, 113
Holland, Isabelle, 16
Hollywood Dream Machine, 20, 81, 117
Homosexual rape, 188–189
Homosexuality, 7–8
   and AIDS, 137, 146, 162, 166
   fiction on, 13, 15–16, 19, 201
   hotline for, 35
   nonfiction on, 21, 23, 162, 166
   organizations for, 33–35
   videocassettes on, 26, 28–29, 32

Homosexuality and Lesbianism: Gay or Straight, Is There a Choice?, 26
Hope Is Not a Method III, 85–86
Hotlines
  for adoption, 134
  for homosexuality, 35
  for sexually transmitted diseases, 178–181
  for unwanted sexual contact, 211
A House for Jonnie O., 112
How To Find Information about AIDS, 163
Hughes, Jean Ogorman, 203
Hyde, Margaret O., 161
Hymen, 40
Hypertonic saline abortions, 98

I Love You, Stupid, 18, 81
I Never Called It Rape: The Ms. Report on Recognizing, Fighting and Surviving Date and Acquaintance Rape, 205
"I Never Thought It Would Be Like This": Teenagers Speak Out about Being Pregnant/Being Parents, 125
I Think I'm Having a Baby, 113, 125
I Want To Keep My Baby, 113
Images and contraceptives, 59
In Love and in Trouble, 116
Incest, 184, 193–194
  in fiction, 197–199
  hotline for, 211
  nonfiction on, 202, 204–205
  organization for, 210–211
Inconvenience and contraceptives, 60
Intercourse, sexual, 6, 41–42
Internal genitals, 39–41
Intrauterine devices, 74–75
Intravenous drug use, AIDS from, 146, 165–166, 174
Irwin, Hadley, 199
Is That What You Want for Yourself?, 125–126

It Only Takes Once, 126
It Won't Happen to Me: Teenagers Talk about Pregnancy, 120
It's OK To Say No Way!, 27, 86
IUDs, 74–75

Jacobs, George, 161
Jelly contraceptives, 68–69, 144, 150
Johnson, Eric W., 21, 51, 82, 162, 203
Johnson, Virginia E., 164
Jones, Elise, 63
Journal of Adolescent Health Care, 55, 89

Kaposi's sarcoma, 145
Keeling, Richard, 169
Kerins, Joseph, 161
Kerr, M. E., 16, 137, 159
Kids Having Kids, 118–119
Kissing, 5
Klein, Norma, 16
Know How, 27
Koertge, Ron, 17, 57, 80, 159
Kolodny, Robert C., 164
Koop, C. Everett, 165
Krumkin, Lyn, 162
Kuklin, Susan, 162
Kurland, Morton L., 162

Lander's Film Review, 24, 52, 84, 123, 167
Langone, John, 163
Lauren, 91–92, 114
Ledray, Linda E., 204
Lee, Joanna, 113
Lee, Mildred, 113
Leonard, John, 162
Lesbians. *See* Homosexuality
Levy, Marilyn, 81, 159, 183, 199
Lice, pubic, 155
Life with Baby, 126
Lingle, Virginia A., 163
Living together, 105
Love & Sex in Plain Language, 21–22, 51, 82–83, 162, 203

Loveletters, 116
Lowry, Lois, 114
Luger, Harriet, 91, 114
Lynda Madaras Talks to Teens about AIDS: An Essential Guide for Parents, Teachers, and Young People, 163

McCoy, Kathy, 22, 43, 52, 120, 164
McGee, Elizabeth, 120
McGuire, Paula, 120
McNaught, Brian, 28
Madaras, Area, 22, 51, 83, 163, 204
Madaras, Lynda, 22, 51, 83, 163–164, 204
Madison, Winifred, 114
Making Decisions about Sex, 27
Making out, 5
Males
  reproductive system of, 38–40
  sexual development of, 42–45
  sexual response of, 3–4
The Man without a Face, 16
March of Dimes, 134
Marriage, 104–105, 115
Masters, William H., 164
Masturbation, 4–5
Maternity homes, 102, 111–112
Matter of Love, 126–127
Mazer, Harry, 18, 81
Mazer, Norma Fox, 18
Me, a Teen Father?, 127
Mecklenburg, Marjorie E., 92
Media Review Digest, 24, 52, 84, 167
Mennonites, homosexual support group for, 34
Menstruation: Hormones in Harmony, 53–54
Menstruation cycle, 41, 46
  and contraception, 63
  fiction about, 49
  nonfiction on, 51
  and pregnancy, 93
  videocassettes on, 53–54

Mi Hermano, 173–174
Michael, Jeannine Masterson, 105, 122
Miklowitz, Gloria D., 114, 136, 159, 183, 199
Miner, Jane Claypool, 121
Miscarriages, 97
Molestation, child, 194
  in fiction, 200
  videocassettes on, 207–208
Mom, I'm Pregnant: A Personal Guide for Teenagers, 122–123
Monseratt, Catherine, 118
Mooney, Elizabeth C., 121
Moore, Kristin A., 121
Mormons, homosexual support group for, 33
Mother, May I?, 127
Mr. and Mrs. Bo Jo Jones, 113
Mucus birth-control method, 63–64
My Darling, My Hamburger, 117
Myths
  about birth control, 77
  videocassettes on, 30, 32

National AIDS Hotline, 179
National Coalition against Sexual Assault (NCASA), 210–211
National Sexually Transmitted Disease Hotline, 179
Neufeld, John, 115
New Teenage Body Book, 22, 43, 52, 120, 164–165
New Ways Ministry, 34–35
NGU (nongonococcal urethritis), 151–152
Night Kites, 16, 137, 159
No Time Soon, 27–28, 86
"Nobody Told Me It Was Rape": A Parent's Guide for Talking with Teenagers about Acquaintance Rape and Sexual Exploitation, 201
Nocturnal emissions, 40
Nonfiction
  on contraception, 81–84
  on physical development, 50–52

Nonfiction (continued)
  on pregnancy, 117–123
  on sexuality, 20–23
  on sexually transmitted diseases, 160–166
  on unwanted sexual contact, 201–206
Nongonococcal urethritis, 151–152
Nonprescription contraceptives, 64–70
Nonprint materials
  on contraception, 84–88
  on physical development, 52–54
  on pregnancy, 123–132
  on sexuality, 23–32
  on sexually transmitted diseases, 167–177
  on unwanted sexual contact, 206–210
Nonspecific urethritis, 151–152
"Not My Daughter": Facing Up to Adolescent Pregnancy, 121
Nourse, Alan E., 165
Novels. See Fiction
NSU (nonspecific urethritis), 151–152
Nugent, Robert, 34

Oettinger, Katherine B., 121
OK To Say No: The Case for Waiting, 28
On Being Gay: A Conversation with Brian McNaught, 28
One Teenager in Ten: Writings by Gay and Lesbian Youth, 21
Open-mouth kissing, 5
Opportunistic diseases, 145
Oral sex, 6
Organizations
  for contraception, 88–89
  for physical development, 54–55
  for pregnancy, 132–134
  for sexually transmitted diseases, 177–178
  for teen sexuality, 33–35
  for unwanted sexual contact, 210–211
Orgasms, 3–4, 42
Orientation, sexual, 6–8
Ours, 133
Ovaries, 41–42
Ovulation, 41–42
  and contraception, 62–64, 75–77

Pap smears, 144
Parasites, 154–156
Parent notification for abortion, 96
Parrot, Andrea, 23, 52, 190, 204
Paul David Silverman Is a Father, 111
Peck, Richard, 115, 200
Pelvic and Breast Examination, 86–87
Pelvic exams, 72, 86–87
Pelvic inflammatory diseases, 75
Penis, 38–39, 42–45
People Who Have Struggled with Abortion, 127–128
Period. See Menstruation cycle
Periodic abstinence, 62–64
Permanent Connections, 14, 57–58, 80
Petting, 5
Philadelphia Gay Switchboard, 35
Phoebe, 111
Physical development, 37
  emotional responses to, 46–47
  in fiction, 49–50
  nonfiction on, 50–52
  nonprint materials on, 52–54
  organizations for, 54–55
  of reproductive systems, 38–41
  sexual, 42–46
  and sexual intercourse, 41–42
PID (pelvic inflammatory disease), 75
Pill, birth-control, 75–77
Pink Triangles: A Study of Prejudice of Lesbians and Gay Men, 28–29

Pittman, Karen, 106
Planned Parenthood Federation of America, Inc., 88, 134
Planned Parenthood v. Danforth, 96
PMS (premenstrual syndrome), 41, 54
PMS Access, 54
PMS Treatment Center, 54
Poverty and pregnancy, 106–107, 124–125, 129
Pregnancy
  choices in, 95–105
  emotional responses to, 94–95
  in fiction, 91, 110–117
  and herpes, 143, 172
  hotlines for, 134
  nonfiction on, 117–123
  nonprint materials on, 123–132
  organizations for, 132–134
  and poverty, 106–107, 124–125, 129
  prevention of. *See* Contraception
  recognizing, 92–94
  role of fathers in, 107–108
  and schooling, 106
  and syphilis, 153
Pregnant Teens: Taking Care, 128
Premenstrual syndrome, 41, 54
Prenatal care, 99–101
Prescription contraceptives, 70–77
Presenting a Personal Safety Curriculum, 208
Pressure
  fiction about, 20
  videocassettes on, 24–25, 27, 126
Prevention of sexually transmitted diseases, 140–141
Prince, Alison, 115
Private adoptions, 103
Private Crisis, Public Cost: Policy Perspectives on Teenage Childbearing, 121
Prostaglandin abortions, 98

Puberty, 42
Pubic lice, 155
Putting Heather Together Again, 81, 159, 183–184, 199

"Questions about AIDS," 166
Questions & Answers on AIDS, 162

Rabble Starkey, 114
Rape, 184, 186–192
  in fiction, 81, 158–159, 198–201
  nonfiction on, 23, 52, 201–206
  organization for, 210–211
  videocassettes on, 206–210
Real People: Meet a Teenage Mother, 128
Recovering from Rape, 204
Religion, 9, 34–35, 60–62
Reproductive systems, 38–41
Research Report for Teenagers: Facts about Sexual Assault, 201–202
Resources
  for contraception, 79–89
  for physical development, 49–55
  for pregnancy, 110–134
  for sexuality, 12–35
  for sexually transmitted diseases, 158–181
  for unwanted sexual contact, 197–211
Responses, sexual, 3–4
Responsibility and contraceptives, 60
Rhythm birth-control method, 62–63
Richards, Arlene Kramer, 106, 121
Risking the Future: Adolescent Sexuality, Pregnancy, and Childbearing, 120
Risks
  in abortions, 99
  in childbirth, 100
Roe v. Wade, 96

222 INDEX

Role models, 6
Rubbers. *See* Condoms
Ruby, Lois, 115
Ruby, 15

Saavedra, Dane, 22, 51, 83, 164, 204
Safe Sex in a Dangerous World: Understanding and Coping with the Threat of AIDS, 165
Saline abortions, 98
Sandler, Bernice R., 203
Saying "No": A Few Words to Young Women about Sex, 29
Scabies, 156
School Library Booklist, 24, 52, 84, 123, 167
Schoolboy Father, 128–129
Schooling and pregnancy, 106
Scoppettone, Sandra, 19, 201
Scrotum, 38–39, 43–44
Secrets Not Meant To Be Kept, 200
Sex and Decisions: Remember Tomorrow, 29
Sex and the American Teenager, 29–30
Sex, Choices and You, 30
Sex, Drugs & AIDS, 165–166, 174
Sex Education, 1–2, 14, 50
Sex Myths and Facts, 30
Sexual Abstinence: The Right Choice?, 87
Sexual Abuse and Harassment: Causes, Prevention...Coping, 208–209
Sexual Responsibility: A Two-Way Street, 30–31
Sexuality
  activities in, 4–6
  expressions of, 3–4
  in fiction, 12–20
  hotlines for, 35
  nonfiction on, 20–23
  nonprint materials on, 23–32
  organizations for, 33–35
  orientation of, 6–8
  shaping of, 2–3
  values and choices in, 8–10

Sexually transmitted diseases, 135–138
  bacteria, 149–154
  and contraception, 59, 63, 66, 68–69, 73–74, 76
  detection of, 139–140
  in fiction, 158–160
  hotlines for, 178–181
  nonfiction on, 160–166
  nonprint materials on, 167–177
  organizations for, 177–178
  parasites, 154–156
  responsibilities for, 140–141
  signs of, 138–139
  viruses, 142–149
Sexually Transmitted Diseases, 174
Sexually Transmitted Diseases: What You Should Know, 174
Sharelle, 115
Sheedy, Ally, 167
Shelley & Pete (...& Carol), 129
Sherburne, Zoa, 116
Shreve, Susan, 116
Siedor, Collin, 209
Single parenting, 105
  in fiction, 112, 114–115
  videocassette on, 123–124
Smart Talk, 175
So Many Voices: A Look at Abortion in America, 129
"So You Think You Might Be Pregnant," 120
Society, influence of, 3, 9
Society for Adolescent Medicine, 55, 89
A Solitary Secret, 198
Someone To Love Me, 112
Someone You Know, 209
Someone You Know: Acquaintance Rape, 209
Sooner or Later? Issues of Teenage Sexuality, 31
Sperm, 39, 41–42
Spermicides, 66–69
Sponge contraceptives, 69–70
Spontaneous abortions, 97
State AIDS hotlines, 179–181

Statutory rape, 186–187
STD. *See* Sexually transmitted
    diseases
STD Blues, 175
*The STD Gang: Prevention and
    Treatment*, 175
Stephensen, A. M., 116
Stereotypes, sexual, 3
Sterility from sexually transmitted
    diseases, 140
Sticks and Stones, 15–16
Stop Date Rape, 209–210
Stranger rape, 187, 198–200
Stranger, You and I, 111
Strasser, Todd, 19, 81
The Subject Is AIDS, 175–176
Suppository contraceptives, 69–70
Supreme Court abortion
    decisions, 96
*Surgeon General's Report on
    Acquired Immune Deficiency
    Syndrome*, 165
Surviving Sexual Assault, 203
Sutherland, Joan, 202
Sweet Sixteen and Never..., 13,
    79, 110
Sycamore Year, 113–114
Synagogues for homosexuals,
    33–34
Syphilis, 152–153

Tanner, J. M., 42–43
Teen Mother—A Story of Coping,
    129–130
Teen Pregnancy, 119
*Teen Pregnancy: The Challenges
    We Faced, the Choices We
    Made*, 119
*Teenage Birth Control: Why
    Doesn't It Work?*, 31, 87
Teenage Father, 130
Teenage Homosexuality, 32
*Teenage Mother: Beyond the Baby
    Shower*, 130
*Teenage Parents, Their Lives
    Have Changed*, 130
Teenage pregnancy. *See*
    Pregnancy

"Teenage Pregnancy: A
    Grandmother Too Soon!," 123
*Teenage Pregnancy: A New
    Beginning*, 118
*Teenage Pregnancy: No Easy
    Answers*, 131
"Teenage Pregnancy: The Crisis in
    America," 123
*The Teenage Pregnancy
    Experience*, 87–88, 131
Teenage Sex: How To Say No, 32
Teens Having Babies, 131
Temperature birth-control
    method, 64
Testicles, 39, 39, 43–44
Testosterone, 43
Tests
    for pregnancy, 93–94
    for sexually transmitted
        diseases, 139–140, 153
Then Again, Maybe I Won't,
    37–38, 49
Thompson, Patricia G., 92
Too Bad about the Haines Girl, 116
*Top Secret: Sexual Assault
    Information for Teenagers
    Only*, 202–203
Touching, 3
Transsexuals, 8
Transvestites, 8
Travelers, 14, 58, 80
Treatment for sexually
    transmitted diseases, 141
Trichomonas vaginalis, 154–155
Trivelpiece, Laurel, 116
Truss, Jan, 117
The Turkey's Nest, 115

Ulene, Art, 165
Unbirthday, 116
*Understanding AIDS: What Teens
    Need To Know*, 176
*Understanding Human
    Reproduction*, 54
*Understanding Social Issues:
    Abortion*, 122
Unitarian-Universalist Office of
    Lesbian and Gay Concerns, 35

U.S. Public Health Service Public Affairs Office, 178
Unwanted sexual contact, 183–184
  abuse, 192–195
  assault, 185–192
  in fiction, 197–201
  hotline for, 211,
  nonfiction on, 201–206
  nonprint materials on, 206–210
  organizations for, 210–211
Unwed Mother, 114–115
Up in Seth's Room, 18–19
Urethra, 39
Urine pregnancy tests, 93–94
Uterus, 40–42
UULGC World, 35

Vacuum aspiration abortions, 97
Vagina, 40–42
Vaginal sexual intercourse, 6, 41–42
Values, 8–10
Van Gelder, Lindsy, 123
VDRL blood tests, 153
Venereal disease. See Sexually transmitted diseases
Venereal warts, 148–149
A Very Delicate Matter, 176
The Very Last Virgin at Hobeck High, 20
A Very Touchy Subject, 19, 81
Video Source Book, 24, 52, 84, 167
Videocassettes
  on contraception, 84–88
  on physical development, 52–54
  on pregnancy, 123–132
  on sexuality, 23–32
  on sexually transmitted diseases, 167–177
  on unwanted sexual contact, 206–210
Vinovskis, Maris A., 122
Viruses, 142–149
Vulva, 40

Wachter, Oralee, 165
Walters, Barbara, 168
Ward, Elizabeth, 205
Warshaw, Robin, 186, 205
Warts, venereal, 148–149
Westheimer, Ruth, 30
Weston, Carol, 23, 83, 122, 166, 206
Wet dreams, 40, 49
Wharton, Mandy, 122
What Do You Do in Quicksand?, 115–116
What To Do If You or Someone You Know Is under 18 and Pregnant, 121–122
What We Need To Know about AIDS Now!: The AIDS File, 161
What You Don't Know CAN kill You: Sexually Transmitted Diseases and AIDS, 176–177
The What's Happening to My Body? Book for Boys: A Growing Up Guide for Parents and Sons, 22, 51–52, 83, 164, 204
The What's Happening to My Body? Book for Girls: A Growing Up Guide for Parents and Daughters, 22, 51, 83, 163–164, 204
When Teens Get Pregnant, 132
Where the Kissing Never Stops, 17–18, 57–58, 80
Why Am I So Miserable If These Are the Best Years of My Life?: Everything Your Mother Never Told You about Becoming a Woman, 21, 50–51, 82, 119, 161, 202
Why Me? The Story of Jenny, 158, 198
Wibbelsman, Charles, 22, 43, 52, 120, 164
Williams, Grace, 20
Willis, Irene, 106, 121
Without Consent, 210

Witt, Reni L., 105, 122
Wittet, Scott, 206
Wong, Debbie, 206
Woods, M. Sandra, 163

Yeast infections, 153–154
You Can Do Something about AIDS, 160

You Would If You Loved Me: Making Decisions about Sex, 32
Young Fathers: Teenage Love, 132
Young Parents, 121
Young, Proud and Gay!, 23, 166

Zindel, Bonnie, 20, 81, 117
Zindel, Paul, 117